Instructor's Manual and Testbank to Accompany

# NURSING IN TODAY'S WORLD

## CHALLENGES, ISSUES, AND TRENDS

### Sixth Edition

W9-CNC-653

Instructor's Manual and Testbank to Accompany

# NURSING IN TODAY'S WORLD

## CHALLENGES, ISSUES, AND TRENDS

### Sixth Edition

**Janice Rider Ellis, PhD, RN**
Professor and Director of Nursing Education
Shoreline Community College
Seattle, Washington

**Celia Love Hartley, MN, RN**
Professor and Chairperson, Health Sciences Division
Director, Nursing Programs
College of the Desert
Palm Desert, California

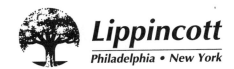

*Lippincott*
*Philadelphia • New York*

| *Ancillary Editor:* | Doris S. Wray |
| *Acquisition Editor:* | Lisa Marshall |
| *Assistant Publisher:* | Sandra Kasko |
| *Compositor:* | JR Bidwell/Tactical Graphics |
| *Printer/Binder:* | R.R. Donnelley & Sons Company/Crawfordsville |

Sixth edition

ISBN: 0-7817-1493-1

Any procedure or practice described in this book should be applied by the health care practitioner under appropriate supervision in accordance with professional standards of care used with regard to the unique circumstances that apply in each practice situation. Care has been taken to confirm the accuracy of information presented and to describe generally accepted practices. However, the authors, editors, and publisher cannot accept any responsibility for errors or omissions or for any consequences from application of the information in this book and make no warranty, express or implied, with respect to the contents of the book. Every effort has been made to ensure drug selections and dosages are in accordance with current recommendations and practice. Because of ongoing research, changes in government regulations, and the constant flow of information on drug therapy, reactions, and interactions, the reader is cautioned to check the package insert for each drug for indications, dosages, warnings, and precautions, particularly if the drug is new or infrequently used.

# PREFACE

The profession of nursing has undergone major changes in recent years that have resulted in the nurses' role taking on many varying dimensions. Likewise nursing education has experienced a variety of changes. As hospitals have moved to include consumers in a greater part of their care, nursing educators are developing a wide variety of teaching/learning strategies that expand on the traditional lecture mode and require more participation by the student. Faculty members have found that students learn best when they are involved in the learning. The increasing number of adult learners has also challenged nurse educators to examine their established teaching methodologies. Thus, new strategies of learning have emerged. Additionally, the curricula of most nursing programs today place a strong emphasis on critical decision making to assist students who will move into a world of employment that extends into many unstructured settings.

It is with this in mind that the Instructor's Manual has been developed for use with the 6th edition of *Nursing in Today's World: Challenges, Issues, and Trends.* Our goal in developing this Instructor's Manual is to facilitate the instruction and evaluation of the content related to the profession of nursing. We believe it is critical that nurses have an understanding of the circumstances and events that have shaped the profession of nursing as we know it.

In the Instructor's Manual you will find all the traditional methods of evaluating student learning that have been present in earlier editions. You will also find a new section titled "Gaming Strategies."

Each chapter of this manual corresponds with a chapter in the textbook. A statement of purpose provides a review of the major content covered in the chapter. The objectives and key terms repeat those included at the beginning of each textbook chapter and are intended to provide easy reference for the instructor. In some chapters the key terms appear quite long, in others, rather brief. For example, one would naturally expect a longer list of terms for chapters related to legal implications or bioethical considerations.

A variety of test situations are presented next. They are developed in several different formats so that the instructor may select those that best meet the needs of a particular program. If the content is integrated throughout the program, test questions that best fit with other evaluative strategies may be selected. You will also notice that each question is keyed to a particular objective of the chapter. This is intended to facilitate "teaching by objectives" and "testing by objectives." If the content is integrated, this should also assist with the selection of specific topics and the corresponding test questions. In each chapter you will find the following.

**Critical thinking exercises.** Critical thinking, as we use it here, is the process by which an individual analyzes and synthesizes material from multiple sources from an evaluative viewpoint. Logically completed, it results in a clearer, more precise, more significant, and insightful answer that has looked analytically at all possibilities before selecting the best. We see this process as tantamount to good nursing practice today; thus we provide situations that will give students the opportunity to practice the skill. These exercises, while essentially designed to evaluate learning, could also be used in the classroom to stimulate discussion. Groups or individuals might be assigned the various questions to present, defend, or otherwise discuss.

**Discussion/essay questions.** These questions can be used in a number of ways. First, they can be used to direct the discussion that would occur in a seminar-format class. In this sense, they can also be used as preparation for a credit-by-examination test if an instructor deems it appropriate to make that option available to students. Questions selected from this section might also be used appropriately for take-home examinations or as regular midterm or end-of-the-term examinations. These questions also are easily adapted to the concept of pretests in which students are given questions that they are to bring back to the next class session answered as a "ticket to class." This strategy encourages students to come to class prepared to discuss the assigned reading.

**Fill in the blanks.**  Fill-in-the-blank questions offer the advantage of rather typically conforming to the content as presented in the chapter. Because of this they can easily be used in workbook format, as a "ticket to class," for self-study purposes by the students, or for group work in the classroom.

**True-false questions.**  True-false questions offer another method of assessing a student's comprehension of material. They can be used simply as presented or students can be required to apply aspects of critical thinking to the questions by explaining why the answer is true or why it is false. If false, they can be asked to correct it so that it is a true statement. Used in this way these types of questions also provide good material to be assigned for a "ticket to class."

**Matching questions.**  Matching questions offer yet another form of evaluating learning. More than that, they can be used as a study guide for students or can be incorporated into the general testing of content. Matching questions lend themselves to the assessment of basic knowledge with the beginning learner and are particularly useful in evaluating the understanding of key terms and specific language used in health care. They can also be used to assess understanding of relationships.

**Multiple-choice questions.**  This form of testing is popular, because it is the format currently used in licensing examinations. You will note that there are often several questions that address a particular objective or, more specifically, a particular concept. This is intended to allow the instructor to select a wording that best matches his or her class emphasis. It also allows the instructor to develop different, yet equivalent, examinations in instances where the course is taught each term, where more than one section is taught each term, or in situations in which test security is a problem. Multiple-choice testing is easily adapted to grading machines. The possible choices we have offered might also be altered to reflect the emphasis developed in a particular course.

**Gaming in the classroom.**  This type of question is new to this edition and represents one example of the current trend toward using "gaming" in the classroom. For each chapter, categories of topics have been identified that reflect sections of content. Within each category is a series of answers for which the student must provide the questions. Different point values can be assigned depending on the difficulty of the questions. The questions can be used in the classroom in a situation in which students form teams that compete against one another, answers being provided by the group or by individuals in the group. Or the classroom might be divided in half, with one side of the classroom competing with the other for the most points. The questions can also be used for purposes of content review in which interactive participation of students is desired.

We hope this manual will assist and facilitate your instruction. As with the major textbook, your suggestions for change or improvement are always welcomed. If you have thought of other creative ways to use this manual, please share them with us also.

*Janice Rider Ellis, RN, PhD*

*Celia Love Hartley, RN, MN*

# Contents

# 1

# Understanding the Health Care Environment

## PURPOSE

This chapter introduces the student to the major health care agencies in which nurses practice. A general overview of the types of agencies and their differences and similarities will help the student to understand the clinical environments they will be entering. The second major section of this chapter introduces all of the colleagues in health care with whom they may be working. The increasing emphasis on interdisciplinary approaches to client care require that each individual have an understanding of the role that others may play in the individual client's health care plan. Building respect and a collaborative approach will assist the student in adapting to the health care environment. A third component of this chapter is an introduction to the whole arena of alternative and complementary care resources. As more people seek alternatives to high technology and invasive medical care, health care workers need information to interact in positive ways with clients. Through understanding the client's point of view and developing an openness to combining therapeutic approaches, today's health care worker may support the client toward health in a variety of ways.

## OBJECTIVES

1. Discuss the three ways that health care agencies are classified.

2. Describe the various health care settings, including the types of services offered and the roles that registered nurses perform in each.

3. Describe the health care delivery provided in ambulatory care settings and in community agencies.

4. Discuss the roles and interrelationships of the various health care providers in the health care system.

5. Analyze the various issues related to individual health care occupations.

6. Describe the various avenues for alternative health care and analyze their relationship to traditional medical care.

## KEY TERMS

Acute care facility
Alternative health care
Community mental health centers
Complementary therapy
Herbal medicine
Homeopathy
Long-term care facility

Naturopathy
Nonprofit
Nursing home
Osteopathy
Primary care provider
Proprietary agency
Subacute care
Tertiary care hospital
Transitional care

## SITUATIONS TO FOSTER CRITICAL THINKING

1. The change in the way health care delivery is organized has affected the classification of health care agencies. What accreditation concerns would be present if your acute ambulatory care clinic becomes part of the local acute care hospital? (Objective 1)

2. What are the differences and similarities in the nursing roles in ambulatory care settings and hospitals or nursing homes that you have had contact with? (Objective 2)

3. An acute care hospital is opening a sub-acute care unit designed to care for individuals who are expected to need care for 15 to 90 days after their acute hospital stay. These individuals are expected to be discharged home. If you are asked to work on this unit, what questions should you ask about staffing patterns, care delivery approach, accountability and responsibility, and relationships with the rest of the facility? What questions should you ask regarding your own status as an employee? (Objective 2)

4. Changes have occurred in the types of care taking place in ambulatory care settings, and this has affected nurses working in those settings. If you had been working in ambulatory care for 8 years and the agency decided to perform day procedures using intravenous sedation, what questions and concerns should you discuss with your manager?(Objective 3)

5. A multidisciplinary team for a home care agency may be led by the nurse, the physical therapist, or the social worker. Develop a set of criteria that could be used by the agency to determine which professional should be the team leader for an individual client. (Objective 4)

6. Most of the proposals for a reformed health care system involve greater use of a primary care physician as a "gatekeeper" to specialist care. What are the benefits to the system of this approach? What are the problems associated with this approach? Weighing the benefits and problems, take and support a position for or against the use of the primary physician as a "gatekeeper." (Objective 5)

7. Outline the advantages and disadvantages of licensing all individuals who perform the various diagnostic procedures. How would it change relationships in the health care system if a license were not required to perform these procedures? (Objective 5)

8. Consider a situation in which you are caring for a person who has just been diagnosed with cancer. This client confides in you that she plans to seek vitamins or herbs that will cure her and not give her all those awful effects she has seen in others. What will be your course of action and why? (Objective 6)

9. A patient asks you what alternative therapy might be useful in controlling his chronic back pain. How will you respond to this question? What concerns should you address as you talk with the patient? (Objective 6)

## DISCUSSION/ESSAY QUESTIONS

1. What are three ways that health care agencies are classified? (Objective 1)

2. What is the expected length of stay in an acute care hospital? (Objective 1)

3. What is the expected length of stay in a short-stay unit? (Objective 1)

4. Why might a hospital that was traditionally an acute care hospital, open a short-stay unit? (Objective 1)

5. What is the expected length of stay in a long-term care facility? (Objective 1)

6. How does a community hospital differ from a tertiary hospital? (Objective 1)

7. What best characterizes the community hospital? (Objective 1)

8. How do community health agencies differ from traditional public health departments? (Objective 1)

9. How does being a nonprofit agency affect the use of income received from clients and third-party payers? (Objective 1)

10. What factor defines a health care agency as proprietary? (Objective 1)

11. How does a nonprofit agency raise capital funds? (Objective 1)

12. Why was nursing education originally focused in acute care hospitals? (Objective 2)

13. Why were graduates of nursing education programs in the past expected to spend one or more years working in an acute care hospital before working in another setting? (Objective 2)

14. How does a home health care agency differ from a public health department? (Objective 2)

15. How does inpatient care differ from outpatient care? (Objective 2)

16. What are the major differences in resources found in critical or intensive care units as opposed to general medical-surgical units? (Objective 2)

17. What nursing roles might be found in diagnostic units in a hospital? (Objective 2)

18. What responsibilities do nurses in long-term care have that are not a common part of nursing in an acute care hospital? (Objective 2)

19. What types of care services are provided by home care agencies? (Objective 3)

20. In what ways might a newly developed unit, such as a day treatment unit for chemotherapy, offer opportunities for creativity in nursing? (Objective 3)

21. How does assisted living differ from nursing home care? (Objective 3)

22. What is a continuing care retirement community and how does it differ from a nursing home? (Objective 3)

23. How does funding for assisted living differ from funding for nursing home care? (Objective 3)

24. How might changes in Medicare reimbursement for health professional education in hospitals affect the supply of health care providers? (Objective 4)

25. List at least three different occupations that could be considered primary health care providers and explain why you included them. (Objective 4)

26. Discuss the differences between the physician's assistant and the nurse practitioner. (Objective 4)

27. Why are some physicians opposed to nurse practitioners? (Objective 4)

28. Identify a health occupation in which there are both technologists and technicians and explain the education and responsibilities of each. (Objective 4)

29. Identify a health occupation in which there are both therapists and therapy technicians and explain the education and responsibilities of each. (Objective 4)

30. What is the significance of a physician being *board certified*? (Objective 4)

31. In what situations might it not be appropriate for an interdisciplinary care team to be led by a registered nurse? Explain your answer. (Objective 4)

32. Where are shortages of primary care providers most apparent and why? (Objective 5)

33. What are the reasons a person might consult a folk medicine healer rather than a conventional health care provider? (Objective 6)

34. Give an example of an alternative health care approach that might be used to treat a stress-related illness. Why would this approach have the potential for success? (Objective 6)

35. What is the basis of treatment by chiropractors? What types of health problems are most often referred to chiropractors? (Objective 6)

36. What is meant by complementary therapy? (Objective 6)

# FILL IN THE BLANKS

*Instructions: Complete the following statements by filling in the blanks with the word or words that make the sentence complete and correct.*

1. Three ways of classifying health care agencies are according to

   _____, _____, and _____. (Objective 1)

2. Three categories within the length of stay classification are _____, _____, and _____. (Objective 1)

3. Acute care refers to the care commonly given in _____. (Objective 1)

4. The average length of stay in a long-term care facility is _____ to _____. (Objective 1)

5. Short-stay units typically care for patients for less than _____. (Objective 1)

6. A hospital that serves as a referral center for those with complex problems is called _____ care hospital. (Objective 1)

7. Another term for subacute care is _____ care. (Objective 1)

8. Investor-owned health care facilities are termed _____. (Objective 1)

9. An outpatient stays in a hospital less than _____. (Objective 1)

10. A unit that cares for individuals after they leave a critical care unit but still need high-level monitoring is often referred to as a _____ unit. (Objective 2)

11. The agency that is usually responsible for monitoring and maintaining the health of the general population is the _____ _____ _____. (Objective 2)

12. A unit in which people receive chemotherapy or other specific nursing services is often referred to as a

    _____ _____ unit. (Objective 2)

13. The average age of clients in nursing homes is _____. (Objective 2)

14. A facility in which a person may receive help in performing activities of daily living but no health care services is termed an _____ _____ facility. (Objective 2)

15. A retirement center that provides independent living, assisted living, and nursing home care within one organization is referred to as a _____ _____ _____. (Objective 2)

16. A condition that needs care within a short time frame but is not an emergency is often termed an _____ condition. (Objective 3)

17. A setting in which many nurses are hired to supervise staff rather than provide direct care is _____ clinic. (Objective 3)

18. Public health nurses responsible for community health issues are required to have a _____ degree. (Objective 3)

19. Hospice care usually includes management of pain, nausea, anorexia, and other such problems. This is referred to as _____ management. (Objective 3)

20. A problem for those needing mental health services in the community is the lack of adequate _____. (Objective 3)

21. A major change in primary care has been the increase in _____ practice and the decrease in _____ practice. (Objective 4)

22. A health care professional who provides initial entry into the health care delivery system is called a _____ _____ _____ . (Objective 4)

23. Traditional osteopathic medicine included a greater emphasis on _____ _____ and _____ _____ than traditional allopathic medicine. (Objective 4)

24. The official credential that identifies a physician who has completed a specialization residency and an examination requirement is _____ _____. (Objective 4)

25. A podiatrist is authorized to perform surgery on _____. (Objective 4)

26. The eye care professional authorized to treat all diseases of the eye as well as provide services to correct vision is the _____. (Objective 4)

27. Speech therapists are currently required to complete a _____ degree. (Objective 4)

28. The highest-level title among those working in allied health fields is usually _____ . (Objective 4)

29. Some people have suggested that nurse practitioners not be independently licensed but instead be considered _____ _____ . (Objective 5)

30. There is a shortage of physicians in _____ and _____ areas of the United States. (Objective 5)

31. Current data suggests that there are too many _____ physicians. (Objective 5)

32. The Pew Commission Report suggests that professionals prepared as _____ rather than _____ are needed. (Objective 5)

33. The Pew Commission Report suggests that an _____ focus rather than a professional specific focus is needed. (Objective 5)

34. The Pew Commission Report stated that the multiple entry and multiple exit points in nursing education was a _____. (Objective 5)

35. The Pew Commission recommended decreasing the number of schools preparing _____ and _____. (Objective 5)

36. One reason people seek out alternative health care providers is the _____ nature of the interactions these individuals maintain. (Objective 6)

37. Two examples of the therapeutic benefits of nutrients are _____ and _____. (Objective 6)

38. The Agency for Health Care Policy and Research recommends _____ treatment as a useful option. (Objective 6)

39. The naturopath treats disease through _____, _____, _____, _____, and _____. (Objective 6)

40. Major issues in regard to the use of alternative therapies are _____ _____, _____ _____, and principles of _____ and _____. (Objective 6)

## TRUE-FALSE QUESTIONS

*Instructions: Mark the following statements "T" if true or "F" if false. If using a scoring card, mark "A" if true or "B" if false.*

_____ 1. Hospitals are generally classified as acute care facilities. (Objective 1)

_____ 2. A hospital may include both short-term and long-term care components in its services. (Objective 1)

_____ 3. All hospitals are nonprofit organizations. (Objective 1)

_____ 4. Nonprofit hospitals only charge for their costs of providing care. (Objective 1)

_____ 5. Another name for profit making is proprietary. (Objective 1)

_____ 6. Community health agencies commonly provide long-term care. (Objective 1)

_____ 7. The average length of stay in acute care has been shortened since the implementation of diagnosis-related groups. (Objective 1)

_____ 8. Nursing homes are the only entities authorized to provide long-term care. (Objective 1)

_____ 9. Long-term mental health care is only available in state hospitals. (Objective 1)

_____ 10. Subacute care is located only in long-term care facilities. (Objective 1)

_____ 11. A health care facility is classified as governmental if any of its support comes through tax dollars. (Objective 1)

_____ 12. Most nursing homes are nonprofit agencies. (Objective 1)

_____ 13. Most hospitals are nonprofit agencies. (Objective 1)

_____ 14. If a patient stays as long as 24 hours in the hospital, that patient is automatically an inpatient. (Objective 2)

_____ 15. Most hospitals provide diagnostic services only for those admitted to the hospital. (Objective 2)

_____ 16. Some individuals are admitted to a hospice unit for a brief stay to manage symptoms. (Objective 2)

_____ 17. Residents of nursing homes are all expected to live their remaining lives in the facility. (Objective 2)

_____ 18. Salaries for resident physicians are partly subsidized by Medicare funds. (Objective 2)

_____ 19. A tertiary care center focuses on terminal care of the dying patient. (Objective 2)

_____ 20. Physicians are expected to visit their patients in nursing homes on a weekly basis. (Objective 2)

_____ 21. Public health departments are agencies of the government. (Objective 3)

_____ 22. Most public health departments focus on meeting health needs that affect the entire community. (Objective 3)

_____ 23. Home care agencies provide only nursing services. (Objective 3)

_____ 24. Those with mental health problems have a more successful return to employment and family relationships when treated within their own community. (Objective 3)

_____ 25. Day care centers for the elderly focus exclusively on caring for those with cognitive impairment. (Objective 3)

_____ 26. Community mental health agencies are able to meet the needs of all persons with mental illness who do not need hospitalization. (Objective 3)

_____ 27. Resident physicians are fully qualified and licensed to practice medicine. (Objective 4)

_____ 28. In the past the majority of nurses were employed in acute care settings. (Objective 4)

_____ 29. Only a physician can be a primary health care provider. (Objective 4)

_____ 30. Only a doctor of medicine is considered a physician. (Objective 4)

_____ 31. Physicians have a minimum of 8 years of postsecondary education. (Objective 4)

_____ 32. Nurse practitioners have prescriptive authority in all states. (Objective 4)

_____ 33. Optometrists are allowed to diagnose and treat eye disease as well as prescribing corrective lenses. (Objective 4)

_____ 34. The terms *technician* and *technologist* have a legally established meaning. (Objective 4)

_____ 35. Nurse practitioners are unable to charge high enough fees to pay for malpractice insurance if it costs them as much as it costs physicians. (Objective 5)

_____ 36. The Pew Commission Report suggested closing all associate degree nursing programs. (Objective 5)

_____ 37. The Pew Commission Report recommended that all licensure be dropped. (Objective 5)

_____ 38. The Pew Commission Report suggested that some aspects of the health care workforce education system need to be redesigned. (Objective 5)

_____ 39. The Pew Commission identified interdisciplinary skills as an essential component of health professional education. (Objective 5)

_____ 40. The Pew Commission identified that there is a shortage of physicians. (Objective 5)

_____ 41. The most powerful group in the health care system has traditionally been the physicians. (Objective 5)

_____ 42. Alternative health care resources have clearly been shown to provide no objective improvement in any person's health status. (Objective 6)

_____ 43. Relaxation techniques have been shown to be ineffective for real pain or disease. (Objective 6)

_____ 44. One reason for the popularity of alternative health care approaches is that they are often provided in a warm, caring environment. (Objective 6)

_____ 45. The federal government is now funding some research relative to the effectiveness of alternative health care strategies. (Objective 6)

_____ 46. Chiropractic care is currently recommended by the AHCPR as effective in some instances of acute back pain. (Objective 6)

# MATCHING QUESTIONS

*Instructions: Match the numbered items with the most appropriate lettered items.*

## Group A (Objectives 1 and 2)

_____ 1. Hospital that treats uncommon or very complex conditions on a referral basis.

_____ 2. Agency that provides care for the dying person.

_____ 3. Facility that is owned and operated by a profit-making corporation.

_____ 4. Setting that provides for inpatient care after hospitalization for the purpose of rehabilitation.

    a. Transitional care unit

    b. Proprietary facility

    c. Tertiary care center

    d. Hospice

## Group B (Objectives 1 and 2)

_____ 1. Nursing home

_____ 2. Community hospital

_____ 3. Ambulatory surgery center

_____ 4. Profit-making facility

    a. Short-term care facility

    b. Long-term care facility

    c. Acute care facility

    d. Proprietary facility

## Group C (Objective 4)

_____ 1. Primary care provider

_____ 2. Individuals with only a few weeks education.

_____ 3. Individuals who examine vision and prescribe glasses.

_____  4.  Nonphysicians who are independently licensed and have prescriptive authority in some states.

    a. Certified nursing assistants

    b. Physicians, dentists, and nurse practitioners

    c. Optometrist

    d. Nurse practitioners

## Group D (Objective 6)

_____  1.  Chiropractic

_____  2.  Naturopathy

_____  3.  Homeopathy

_____  4.  Reflexology

    a. Massage of the feet to produce relaxation and systemic effect.

    b. Manipulation of the spine to create changes in health status.

    c. Treatment of illness by using very small amounts of substances that cause the problem.

    d. Treatment of illness through the use of diet, exercise, lifestyle management, herbs, and other nonpharmacological means.

## MULTIPLE-CHOICE QUESTIONS

*Instructions: Choose the one best answer for each question.*

1.  What are nursing homes and convalescent centers?

    a. Acute care facilities

    b. Community health care facilities

    c. Alternative health care facilities

    d. Long-term care facilities

    (Objective 1)

2.  How are hospitals classified?

    a. Acute care facilities

    b. Community health care facilities

    c. Alternative health care facilities

    d. Long-term care facilities

    (Objective 1)

3.  How is a public health department classified?

    a. Acute care facilities

    b. Community health care facilities

    c. Alternative health care facilities

    d. Long-term care facilities

    (Objective 1)

4.  What is the length of stay in a conventional hospital?

    a. Short term

    b. Intermediate term

    c. Long term

    d. Any of the above depending on the unit

    (Objective 1)

5.  How is a hospital owned by stockholders classified?

    a. Proprietary

    b. Nonprofit

    c. Community

    d. Tertiary

    (Objective 1)

6.  What do nonprofit hospitals do with profits?

    a. They provide more charitable care.

    b. They reinvest it into the institution.

    c. They provide returns to the community.

    d. They pay higher salaries to employees.

    (Objective 1)

7. Which of the following applies to the average length of stay in an acute care hospital?

a. Growing shorter

b. Growing longer

c. Mandated by law

d. Regulated by insurance coverage

(Objective 2)

8. Which type of agency would provide for physical therapy in the home?

a. Public health department

b. Long-term care facility

c. Ambulatory care facility

d. Home health care agency

(Objective 2)

9. Where are rehabilitation services provided?

a. A hospital

b. A special rehabilitation center

c. A long-term care facility

d. All of the above

(Objective 2)

10. How do most hospitals define an outpatient?

a. A person who stays less than 24 hours

b. A person who stays less than 12 hours

c. A person who stays less than 4 hours

d. A person who leaves immediately

(Objective 2)

11. Which of the following describes a hospitality unit?

a. Provides a place for family to stay with a patient without cost

b. Serves as a waiting area for families during procedures

c. Provides health information and resources to the community

d. Provides a hotel-like place for patients and families to stay before, during, and after treatments

(Objective 2)

12. What is a center that provides gastro-esophago-duodenoscopy, cytoscopy, and colonoscopy called?

a. Imaging center

b. Radiologic unit

c. Endoscopy unit

d. X-ray unit

(Objective 2)

13. Who comprise the majority of long-term care residents?

a. Those who need rehabilitation

b. Those who are developmentally disabled

c. Those who are mentally ill

d. Those who are elderly and unable to manage self-care

(Objective 2)

14. What differentiates a nursing home from an assisted living facility is that a nursing home provides what service not provided by the assisted living facility?

a. Skilled nursing care

b. Support for up to three personal activities of daily living

c. Support for all instrumental activities of daily living

d. Referral to other care sources

(Objective 2)

15. What is the health care institution charged with the responsibility of maintaining the health of the community as a whole?

a. Community mental health center

b. Public health department

c. Visiting nurse agency

d. Health maintenance organization

(Objective 3)

16. Which of the following statements is true of long-term care facilities?

    a. They must all have accreditation.

    b. They include nursing homes and centers for developmentally disabled adults.

    c. They care for persons with acute episodes of chronic illness.

    d. They all receive funding from the federal government under Title VI.

    (Objective 3)

17. Which of the following persons furnishes entry into the health care system?

    a. Primary health care provider

    b. Primary nurse

    c. Family practitioner

    d. Referring physician

    (Objective 4)

18. Which of the following best describes primary health care providers?

    a. Persons who furnish entry into the health care system

    b. Persons assigned to a group of patients in the hospital

    c. Physicians called for a consultation

    d. Insurance companies, such as Blue Cross, that help pay medical bills

    (Objective 4)

19. The term *primary health care provider* refers to which of the following?

    a. The type of nursing care given in hospitals

    b. The first physician a patient ever sees

c. A person who furnishes entry into the health care system

d. A health care organization that provides care at a low cost

(Objective 4)

20. Which of the following statements is true of the physician's assistant (PA)?

    a. All PAs must have completed a baccalaureate program.

    b. All PAs must be licensed in the state in which they practice.

    c. All PAs must work under the direction of a physician.

    d. All of the above.

    (Objective 4)

21. Which of the following phrases best describes a technologist?

    a. An individual with good on-the-job training

    b. An individual with baccalaureate preparation

    c. An individual with an associate degree in an allied health field

    d. An individual with postbaccalaureate preparation

    (Objective 4)

22. A master's degree is required of which of the following health occupations?

    a. Speech therapy

    b. Occupational therapy

    c. Registered dietician

    d. Respiratory therapist

    (Objective 4)

23. Which of the following is one of the phenomena exhibited in the health care delivery system in the last 10 to 20 years?

    a. An increase in the incidence of communicable disease

b. A decrease in the incidence of chronic illness

c. An increase in the number of different health occupations

d. A decrease in demand for preventive health services

(Objective 5)

24. What is one of the problems related to nurses working in expanded roles?

a. Whether such nurses should be classified as physician's assistants

b. The problems of third-party payment

c. Credentials required for practice

d. All of the above

(Objective 5)

25. Which group traditionally had the most power in the health care system?

a. Physicians

b. Hospital administrators

c. Insurance companies

d. Governmental agencies

(Objective 5)

26. Where is there still an inadequate supply of primary health care providers?

a. Suburban areas

b. Urban areas

c. Rural areas

d. All of the above

(Objective 5)

27. Which of the following is true of the number of different allied health professions?

a. It is decreasing.

b. It is staying about the same.

c. It is increasing.

d. It is variable from year to year.

(Objective 5)

28. Which of the following did the Pew Commission recommend?

a. Half of all nursing programs be closed

b. All diploma and associate degree programs be closed

c. Roles of variously educated nurses be more clearly differentiated

d. No changes in nursing

(Objective 5)

29. The Pew Commission recommended which of the following?

a. More specialists be prepared

b. More generalists be prepared

c. More physicians of all types be prepared

d. More medical schools open in rural areas

(Objective 5)

30. The Pew Commission identified which two needed changes in health professional education?

a. More scientific background and higher standards

b. Less general education and more specialized education

c. More highly skilled faculty and increased length of education

d. More emphasis on health promotion and a greater interdisciplinary focus

(Objective 5)

31. Which of the following did the Pew Commission NOT identify as concerns regarding legal regulation of health professions?

a. Rigor

b. Standardization

c. Accountability

d. Flexibility

(Objective 5)

32. What is one major factor that may prompt people to seek an alternative health care system?

    a. Lack of money

    b. The belief system of the individual

    c. Unavailability of conventional care alternatives

    d. Pressure from the media

    (Objective 6)

33. Which of the following circumstances would be most likely to result in a person seeking an alternative health care system?

    a. No one in the conventional agencies is able to provide a cure.

    b. A patient believes that no one in the conventional agency cared about him or her as an individual.

    c. The person was informed about potential side effects of medications and treatments.

    d. The family was asked to participate in providing care.

    (Objective 6)

34. Chiropractic is usually considered which of the following?

    a. Acute care

    b. Community health care

    c. Alternative health care

    d. Long-term care

    (Objective 6)

35. Which of the following is an example of a claim about the therapeutic benefits of food that has been substantiated?

    a. Phytochemicals in certain cruciferous vegetables help protect against bowel cancer.

    b. A substance found in apricot pits is an effective antineoplastic agent.

    c. Taking cod liver oil will relieve the joint pain of osteoarthritis.

    d. Taking megadoses of all vitamins will prevent chronic illness.

    (Objective 6)

36. What is the alternative health care that treats through manipulation of the spine?

    a. Reflexology

    b. Chiropractic

    c. Rolfing

    d. Podiatry

    (Objective 6)

37. What is the alternative health care that treats through the use of food, exercise, air, water, sunshine, and some herbs?

    a. Reflexology

    b. Chiropractic

    c. Rolfing

    d. Naturopathy

    (Objective 6)

38. Which of the following is a major concern with herbal medicines that differs from conventional pharmaceuticals?

    a. They are ineffective.

    b. They have side effects.

    c. They do not have standarized doses of active ingredients.

    d. They always contain contaminants.

    (Objective 6)

39. What is one health care problem for which biofeedback is sometimes effective?

    a. Migraine headaches

    b. Peptic ulcers

c. Stroke

d. Depression

(Objective 6)

40. What is the alternative therapy that is particularly useful for children experiencing pain?

a. Massage therapy

b. Reflexology

c. Chiropractic

d. Visualization

(Objective 6)

# GAMING IN THE CLASSROOM

*Instructions: This game involves selecting teams and a host. The teams compete against one another for points. Each game has several subject categories. After teams are determined, a team is chosen to go first and selects a category. The host then poses the answer and the team provides the correct question for that answer. Each question can be awarded the same number of points or more difficult questions may be given heavier point values. (The instructor might determine which questions are more difficult based on the content emphasized in class.) Points are awarded to the team that is the first to signal and give a correct question. If that team is incorrect, the other team may attempt to provide the correct question and receive the points. The length of time allowed for response can be determined by the class or by the instructor. The team with the most points at the end of the game is declared the winner. Teams may be composed of individual students or groups of students. Teams may determine their answers as a team or may take turns answering as individuals.*

## Categories

A. Classifications of Health Care Agencies

B. Types of Care Provided by Health Care Agencies

C. Roles of Health Care Providers

D. Problems Facing Health Care Providers

E. Alternative Health Care Resources

## Answers and Questions

### Category A

A: Nonprofit.

Q: What is the classification of a facility that uses all profits for enhancing the facility or its services?

A: Long-term care.

Q: What is the classification of a nursing home in terms of length of stay?

A: Provides care for less than 24 hours.

Q: What is a short-stay unit?

A: Transitional care.

Q: What is another name for subacute care?

A: Proprietary.

Q: What is the term for a profit-making facility?

### Category B

A: Critical care unit.

Q: In what type of unit would a person with life-threatening injuries be cared for?

A: Assisted living facility.

Q: What is a facility that provides help with three or fewer personal ADLs and support for all instrumental ADLs?

A: Transitional care unit.

Q: What type of unit provides care after acute hospitalization preparing the person for discharge?

A: Public health department.

Q: What agency focuses on the health of the community as a whole?

A: Outpatient.

Q: How would a patient be classified if coming to the agency only for treatment and then returning home for self-care?

A: Continuing care retirement community.

Q: What type of facility provides independent living, assisted living, and nursing home care?

## Category C

A: Board certified.

Q: What is a specialty physician who has completed a specialty residency and passed a qualifying examination called?

A: Gatekeeper.

Q: What is the term for the professional who is responsible for controlling access to the health care system?

A: Optometrist.

Q: What is the health care provider who provides vision care but does not treat diseases of the eye?

A: Podiatrist.

Q: Who is the health care professional who provides care, including surgery, for the feet?

A: Nurse practitioner.

Q: What is the term for an advanced practice nurse who provides primary care?

## Category D

A: Rural areas.

Q: What areas still experience a shortage of physicians?

A: Specialty physicians.

Q: What type of physician is in oversupply?

A: Increased interdisciplinary approaches.

Q: What is a recommendation of the Pew Commission regarding health professional education?

A: Define differentiated practice based on education.

Q: What is a Pew Commission recommendation about nursing?

A: Health promotion.

Q: What is a Pew Commission recommendation for increased focus in all health professionals education?

## Category E

A: Chiropractic.

Q: What is the therapy that treats by spinal manipulation?

A: Phytochemicals.

Q: What are the nutrients that help prevent bowel cancer?

A: Stress-related illnesses.

Q: What types of illness are effectively treated through relaxation training?

A: Naturopath.

Q: What alternative health care provider treats through a combination of diet, exercise, rest, lifestyle modification, and herbs?

A: Visualization.

Q: What is an alternative therapy for assisting children in managing pain?

# 2

# Health Care Finance and Control

## PURPOSE

This chapter helps the student understand the varied aspects of health care finance and control. Finances determine much of what is happening in the health care delivery system in terms of restructuring, job availability, and consumer expectations. Thus understanding the financial aspects of health care helps to reveal who has what kind of control over actions. Access to health care is also of critical concern to nurses and is influenced by economic, geographic, and social factors. Understanding these critical issues will assist the student in functioning more effectively within the system.

## OBJECTIVES

1. Describe different mechanisms for financing health care.

2. Explain how the role of the federal government in health care financing has affected the system.

3. Discuss the various approaches that are being used to manage costs in the health care delivery system including changing patterns of payment and controlling providers.

4. Analyze the issues related to access to health care including types of barriers and indicators of access.

5. Discuss the mechanisms being used to measure and insure quality in organizations and agencies that are delivering health care.

6. Analyze the use of power by regulatory agencies, payers, providers, and consumers in the health care system.

7. Explain continuing concerns regarding effective use of health care and changing the system.

## KEY TERMS

Capitation
Case management
Comorbidity
Cost containment
Diagnosis-related groups (DRGs)
Fee-for-service
Health maintenance organization (HMO)
Insurance
Joint Commission for the Accreditation of Healthcare Organizations (JCAHO)
Key indicators
Long-term care
Managed care
Medicaid
Medicare
Medicare intermediary
Outcome measures
Point-of-service plan
Power
Preferred provider organization (PPO)
Primary care provider
Prospective payment
Quality indicators
Restructuring
Third-party payer
Vertically integrated systems

## SITUATIONS TO FOSTER CRITICAL THINKING

1. Choose a health insurance plan available in your area. Analyze it in relationship to cost, comprehensiveness, choices, and accessibility. (Objective 1)

2. Choose a health maintenance plan in your area. Analyze it in relationship to cost, comprehensiveness, choices, and accessibility. (Objective 1)

3. Identify two or three Medicare supplement plans available in your community. Compare them in terms of cost, comprehensiveness, choices, and accessibility. (Objective 1)

4. Choose a common admission diagnosis in which you have clinical experiences. Investigate the DRG, the average length of stay, the length of stay required for the case to be considered an "outlier," and the reimbursement amount. Compare this with the progress and length of stay of an individual patient. (Objective 3)

5. Investigate the state reimbursement for an "average" nursing home resident who is supported by public assistance. Compare this with the rate charged a privately paying nursing home resident. What do you think might be the consequences of any differences you have identified? (Objective 3)

6. If a health plan reimburses primary care providers based on a capitation system, what will be the effect on income and expenses of a patient who needs frequent care appointments? Analyze how the use of capitation might affect the quality of health care for the individual consumer. (Objective 3)

7. Identify the resources for care for those in your community who do not have health insurance coverage. If they were unable to pay, where could they go for preventive health services? For emergency services? For routine illness care? (Objective 4)

8. Find out your state's immunization rate for infants and preschool children. Compare these with the current CDC recommendations. If there is a discrepancy, identify ways that your student group could assist in improving the immunization rate for this vulnerable group. (Objective 4)

9. Explore the mechanisms for measuring quality of care currently being used in the facility or agency where you have clinical practice. Analyze these mechanisms to identify what areas may not be evaluated using these mechanisms. (Objective 5)

10. If a consumer has a complaint about the health care services provided by an agency in your community, what would you advise that consumer to do in relationship to the perceived poor care and why? (Objective 6)

11. Evaluate the effects of any restructuring that has been done in a health care facility or agency in your community. (Objective 7)

## DISCUSSION/ESSAY QUESTIONS

1. What is a health maintenance organization (HMO)? (Objective 1)

2. What is a preferred provider organization (PPO)? (Objective 1)

3. Identify a PPO in your community. (Objective 1)

4. How does traditional health insurance differ from a managed care plan? (Objective 1)

5. Who is eligible for Medicare? (Objective 2)

6. Who is eligible for Medicaid? (Objective 2)

7. What funding resource will assist the person who has end-stage renal disease and who needs dialysis? (Objective 2)

8. Why are hospital censuses going down in most parts of the country? (Objective 3)

9. What are DRGs and how are they related to the prospective payment system? (Objective 3)

10. What is capitation when used in regard to a health care plan payment? (Objective 3)

11. How have DRGs affected length of stay in acute care hospitals? (Objective 3)

12. What is meant by lack of geographic access to health care services? (Objective 4)

13. What is meant by lack of economic access to health care services? (Objective 4)

14. What is meant by lack of cultural access to health care services? (Objective 4)

15. What factors affect access to health care services? (Objective 4)

16. What is the role of the Joint Commission for the Accreditation of Healthcare Organizations (JCAHO) in measuring and insuring quality in hospitals? (Objective 5)

17. What is the purpose of the Utilization and Quality Control Peer Review Organization (PRO)? (Objective 5)

18. What is the purpose of the Community Health Accreditation Program (CHAP)? (Objective 5)

19. What is the purpose of the National Committee for Quality Assurance (NCQA) Review? (Objective 5)

20. HEDIS data are used to evaluate primarily what aspect of health care? (Objective 5)

21. How is medical practice in hospitals evaluated? (Objective 5)

22. How has the role of the patient/client in the health care system changed over the last 10 years? (Objective 6)

23. What group has traditionally had the most power in the health care system? Do you see any changes in this occurring in your community? If so, describe them. (Objective 6)

24. What constraints are third-party payers putting on physician practice? (Objective 6)

25. How might nurses increase their power in the health care system? (Objective 6)

26. Why is cost containment a major concern in health care? (Objective 7)

27. How does cost containment affect the delivery of nursing care? (Objective 7)

28. Why are hospitals expressing concern about the use of the emergency room for nonemergency conditions? (Objective 7)

29. How are key indicators used to identify effective use of health care resources? (Objective 7)

30. What is a major strength of the United States health care system? (Objective 7)

31. How is the pressure to be cost-effective affecting nursing practice? (Objective 7)

# FILL IN THE BLANKS

*Instructions: Complete the following statements by filling in the blanks with the word or words that make the sentence complete and correct.*

1. Four different mechanisms for financing health care are _____ _____, _____ _____, _____ _____, and _____ _____. (Objective 1)

2. Any entity that pays health care bills for an individual is termed a _____ _____ _____. (Objective 1)

3. One example of charitable care is the _____ _____ that provides care for burned children. (Objective 1)

4. Health insurance plans first began in the _____. (Objective 1)

5. The Blue Cross and Blue Shield organizations were traditionally organized as _____ corporations. (Objective 1)

6. In addition to paying for care, insurance companies also establish _____ for care. (Objective 1)

7. The two major federal programs for financing health care that were developed as a part of the Social Security Act are _____ and _____. (Objective 2)

8. Medicare provides health care primarily for the _____, whereas Medicaid provides health care for the _____. (Objective 2)

9. HMOs that supplement Medicare often result in a loss of _____ for the consumer. (Objective 2)

10. Medicare legislation was one of the first places to officially define _____

nursing. (Objective 2)

11. Medicare and Medicaid were the first payers that mandated _____ in the interests of cost containment. (Objective 2)

12. The military program that reimburses for care in the private sector is _____. (Objective 2)

13. The categories used to determine payment under Medicare are called _____. (Objective 2)

14. A PPO is a _____ _____ _____. (Objective 3)

15. DRG stands for _____ _____ _____. (Objective 3)

16. The payment system that provides a predetermined reimbursement regardless of specific client costs is a _____ _____ _____. (Objective 3)

17. Third-party payers have attempted to control costs through changing patterns of _____. (Objective 3)

18. Third-party payers have attempted to control costs through _____ actions of providers. (Objective 3)

19. When health care is paid for each time a service is provided this is termed _____-_____-_____. (Objective 3)

20. A reimbursement amount for a procedure or illness that has been determined in advance of the provision of service is _____ payment. (objective 3)

21. When calculating a payment for a DRG, the amount is increased when a second illness called a _____ is present. (Objective 3)

22. A person whose hospital stay is significantly longer than the average is termed an _____. (Objective 3)

23. A future goal of some in the Medicare program is to increase the scope of the DRG payment so that it also includes the payment to the _____. (Objective 3)

24. Nursing actions that help to contain costs include preventing _____. (Objective 3)

25. Any system in which the use of health care services is carefully controlled and monitored to ensure that policies are followed is termed _____ _____. (Objective 3)

26. A method that is used to move an individual requiring major health care through the system efficiently is called _____ _____. (Objective 3)

27. To control all aspects of health care, organizations have formed alliances that include providers at each level from primary care through tertiary care as well as the third-party payer. These are called _____ _____ organizations. (Objective 3)

28. Three major categories of barriers to access to health care services are _____, _____, and _____. (Objective 4)

29. The three main focuses for access to health care are _____, _____, and _____. (Objective 4)

30. One barrier to economic access to health care is the _____ in employers who provide health insurance coverage. (Objective 4)

31. _____ _____ areas of cities have fewer health care providers. (Objective 4)

32. Making care culturally accessible for those who speak other languages requires the use of _____. (Objective 4)

33. The organization that accredits hospitals is called the _____. (Objective 5)

34. The National Committee for Quality Assurance (NCQA) accredits _____. (Objective 5)

35. Medicare requires that each hospital contract with an external medical review organization called a _____ and _____ ____ _____ _____ _____. (Objective 5)

36. A standardized tool to monitor outcomes that describes the optimum progression through the system is called a _____ _____. (Objective 5)

37. The health care discipline that has traditionally had the most power in the system is _____. (Objective 6)

38. The power held by the governmental agencies that control health care is termed _____ power. (Objective 6)

39. A major source of financial power in the health care system are _____ _____ _____. (Objective 6)

40. The most costly place to seek routine ambulatory care is the _____ _____. (Objective 7)

41. A specific, measurable aspect of health care that reflects the effectiveness of the system as a whole is called a _____ _____. (Objective 7)

## TRUE-FALSE QUESTIONS

*Instructions: Mark the following statements "T" if true or "F" if false. If using a scoring card, mark "A" if true or "B" if false.*

_____ 1. Organizations that contract to pay health care costs for an individual are referred to as third-party payers. (Objective 1)

_____ 2. Hospitals provide charitable care adequate to meet the health care needs of those who do not have financial resources. (Objective 1)

_____ 3. All hospitals are considered charita-ble, nonprofit organizations. (Objective 1)

_____ 4. Health insurance began in the 1930s in the United States. (Objective 1)

_____ 5. The United States is one of the very few industrialized countries of the world that does not have some type of universal health care coverage for all its residents. (Objective 1)

_____ 6. HMOs (health maintenance organi-zations) were the first third-party payers to pay for preventive health care services. (Objective 1)

_____ 7. When filing claims for Medicare, individuals deal directly with the Social Security Agency. (Objective 1)

_____ 8. The federal government affects only the health care provided through Medicare and Medicaid. (Objective 2)

_____ 9. The federal government has encour-aged the development of health maintenance organizations. (Objective 2)

_____ 10. Medicaid, which funds indigent care, is fully managed by the federal government. (Objective 2)

_____ 11. Part B of Medicare, which funds outpatient and physician costs, is optional for those enrolled in the program. (Objective 2)

_____ 12. Military members and their depen-dents are required to receive all of their care in military hospitals and clinics. (Objective 2)

_____ 13. Most of the increase in costs in health care is due to higher salaries for nurses. (Objective 3)

_____ 14. Health care costs have risen faster than the general rate of inflation for the United States. (Objective 3)

_____ 15. Fee-for-service payment systems have encouraged the provision of more services which generated more income. (Objective 3)

_____ 16. Insurance company reimbursements have more than met the costs of care. (Objective 3)

_____ 17. When an insurance company or Medicare states that it pays 80% of the cost of a service, the consumer can be sure that he or she will only be responsible for 20% of the cost determined by the provider. (Objective 3)

_____ 18. A DRG (diagnosis-related group) is a category of illness that has been determined by the Health Care Financing Administration to require a specified level of reimbursement. (Objective 3)

_____ 19. DRGs were instituted to provide a more equitable distribution of costs between the Medicare program and the consumer. (Objective 3)

_____ 20. In prospective payment systems, the burden of risk is placed on the provider of services. (Objective 3)

_____ 21. When a hospitalized individual has a complicating diagnosis, the hospital will always lose money on care. (Objective 3)

_____ 22. Documentation of care by nurses, especially related to any complication, is essential to effective cost management by health care institutions and agencies. (Objective 3)

_____ 23. DRGs and other cost containment measures have resulted in decreased lengths of hospital stay. (Objective 3)

_____ 24. In a capitated system the provider receives an additional payment whenever a client is hospitalized. (Objective 3)

_____ 25. A preferred provider is so designated because of the high standard of health care services provided. (Objective 3)

_____ 26. Managed care refers only to specific health maintenance organizations that designate providers. (Objective 3)

_____ 27. Most managed care plans rely on a designated "gatekeeper" to prevent excessive use of services. (Objective 3)

_____ 28. Nurses commonly fill the role of case manager. (Objective 3)

_____ 29. An internal case manager is employed by an insurance company to manage care across all areas of care including outpatient and inpatient. (Objective 3)

_____ 30. Acuity measures identify the seriousness of the illness and therefore the resources that will be needed for care. (Objective 3)

_____ 31. Access to health care refers to the ability of the individual to obtain and utilize health care services. (Objective 4)

_____ 32. Economic access refers to the ability to pay for care oneself. (Objective 4)

_____ 33. Economic access is enhanced by making health care policies more comprehensive and providing more liberal benefits. (Objective 4)

_____ 34. A preexisting illness that limits the ability to obtain health insurance decreases economic access to health care services. (Objective 4)

_____ 35. There is less access to health care services in economically depressed areas of large cities. (Objective 4)

_____ 36. When individuals feel uncomfortable in a health care setting because of differences in cultural background, access to health care decreases. (Objective 4)

_____ 37. The federal government provides

the only accreditation of health care agencies. (Objective 5)

_____ 38. Accreditation of a health care agency guarantees the consumer that all standards of care will be met. (Objective 5)

_____ 39. The Joint Commission's accreditation provides an agency with "deemed status" for Medicare and Medicaid. (Objective 5)

_____ 40. Hospitals were first mandated to set up evaluation processes by Medicare legislation. (Objective 5)

_____ 41. If a hospital's statistical outcomes of care are not favorable, the consumer should avoid that hospital because this means care standards are low. (Objective 5)

_____ 42. The clinical pathway ensures that outcomes will be met. (Objective 5)

_____ 43. A major source of power within the health care system is the control of funding. (Objective 6)

_____ 44. Regulatory power in health care is exercised by hospitals. (Objective 5)

_____ 45. Consumers hold most of the financial power in the health care system. (Objective 6)

_____ 46. Nurses have power in the health care system based on collective bargaining and shared governance. (Objective 6)

_____ 47. There are clear indicators that show increased access to reproductive health services by poor women. (Objective 7)

_____ 48. Lack of prenatal care is still a problem among minority women. (Objective 7)

_____ 49. Access to dental health care is even more limited than general health care. (Objective 7)

# MATCHING QUESTIONS

*Instructions: Match the numbered items with the most appropriate lettered items.*

## Group A (Objective 1)

_____ 1. Third-party payer

_____ 2. Medicaid

_____ 3. Health maintenance organization

_____ 4. Managed care

    a. A federal program operated through the states to provide health care for the indigent.

    b. A third-party payer organization that has a major focus on paying for preventive health care services.

    c. An agency or organization that pays for health care received by a consumer.

    d. A program whereby the use of health care services is monitored and controlled.

## Group B (Objective 3)

_____ 1. Capitation

_____ 2. DRG

_____ 3. Comorbidity

_____ 4. PPO

    a. A health care provider that contracts with a third-party payer to provide services at a predetermined, usually lower, rate.

    b. A category used to determine payment under Medicare.

    c. A coexisting or complicating illness in a person who is hospitalized for another diagnosis.

    d. A payment method based on a predetermined fee for each person in the plan.

## Group C (Objective 4)

_____  1. Rural areas

_____  2. Translators

_____  3. Preexisting illness

_____  4. Increasing copayments

     a. A setting in which geographic access to health care is limited.

     b. A condition that contributes to lack of economic access to health care.

     c. A solution to problems of cultural access to health care.

     d. A situation that decreases economic access for those who have health insurance.

## Group D (Objective 5)

_____  1. JCAHO

_____  2. CHAP

_____  3. NCQA

_____  4. HEDIS

     a. A set of statistics that reflect effectiveness of preventive health care services.

     b. An organization that evaluates and accredits hospitals and other health care agencies.

     c. An organization that evaluates and accredits home health care agencies.

     d. An organization that evaluates and accredits health maintenance organizations.

## MULTIPLE-CHOICE QUESTIONS

_Instructions: Match the numbered items with the most appropriate lettered items._

1. If you have a patient aged 85, what program will most likely be paying for health care costs?

   a. Medicare

   b. Medicaid

   c. HCFA

   d. A PPO

   (Objective 1)

2. If your patient is receiving public assistance for living expenses, what program might pay for health care costs?

   a. Medicare

   b. Medicaid

   c. HCFA

   d. A PPO

   (Objective 1)

3. Where have most hospitals obtained the funds to cover the costs of uncompensated care?

   a. Medicaid

   b. Through increased charges to paying clients

   c. Through solicitation of community donations

   d. From charitable and religious organizations

   (Objective 1)

4. If you are working with an individual on Medicare who was denied payment for the rehabilitation visits, what should you recommend?

   a. Submit the claim to Medicaid for payment.

b. Seek a community agency to provide free care.

c. Appeal the Medicare denial.

d. Develop a personal rehabilitation program that does not require health provider supervision.

(Objective 1)

5. All EXCEPT which of the following are solely federal programs for paying for health care services?

a. CHAMPUS

b. Medicaid

c. Medicare

d. Indian Health Service

(Objective 1)

6. Health insurance plans do which of the following?

a. Cover almost all residents of the United States

b. Pay for all health care costs for those who are insured

c. Are required to accept any applicant for insurance

d. Endeavor to limit their risk and maximize profits

(Objective 1)

7. What is one of the major benefits that health maintenance organizations offer over other health care providers?

a. They are more personal.

b. They tend to emphasize preventive care.

c. They are all well located for availability to all.

d. The client can always have a choice of care providers.

(Objective 1)

8. Who initiated evaluation of health care services?

a. Organizations of health care providers

b. Medicare

c. State governments

d. Hospitals

(Objective 2)

9. Which organization or plan defined skilled nursing in its basic reimbursement plan?

a. Medicare

b. Preferred provider organizations (PPOs)

c. Health maintenance organizations (HMOs)

d. Joint Commission (JCAHO)

(Objective 2)

10. Why has the federal government encouraged the development of HMOs?

a. HMOs were one of the earliest plans to manage care.

b. The government is concerned with preventive services.

c. HMOs had a strong history of cost containment.

d. The government wanted to enhance competition in health care.

(Objective 2)

11. Where did the use of a prospective payment system originate?

a. Medicare

b. Group health insurance

c. Health maintenance organizations

d. Preferred provider organizations

(Objective 2)

12. For which group does the federal government provide direct health care services rather than reimbursing for health care obtained in the private sector?

    a. Veterans

    b. Medically indigent

    c. Military dependents

    d. Public health service members

    (Objective 2)

13. Which of the following statements accurately expresses the current status of health planning and resources development?

    a. Federal support is available for local areas willing to match funds.

    b. Federal support is available without the need for matching funds locally.

    c. Federal support takes the form of advisers who work with local agencies.

    b. There is no federal support for health planning and resources development.

    (Objective 2)

14. Which of the following federal programs provides for care in renal failure?

    a. Medicare

    b. The Health Planning and Utilization Act

    c. Medicaid

    d. There is no federal assistance for chronic renal dialysis.

    (Objective 2)

15. What is Medicaid?

    a. A federal program administered by the participating individual states

    b. A federal program administered by the United States Health Department

    c. A state program entirely financed and directed by states

    d. A federal program administered by local governmental agencies

    (Objective 2)

16. Which of the following is a major contributor to health care costs?

    a. Nurses' salary increases

    b. New technology

    c. Increased lengths of hospital stay

    d. The high cost of required immunizations for children

    (Objective 3)

17. Which health cost factor do nurses in acute care have the most ability to affect?

    a. Length of stay

    b. Technologies ordered

    c. Pharmaceutical costs

    d. Salaries of health care workers

    (Objective 3)

18. What is a major problem creating economic loss for acute care hospitals?

    a. The high cost of renal dialysis

    b. The increasing elderly population

    c. Uncompensated care

    d. Pressure for new technology

    (Objective 3)

19. What is the most important cause of increases in the cost of health care?

    a. The effect of raises in nurses' salaries

    b. The fact that the average patient's stay in the hospital is shorter

    c. The cost of new technology

    d. The increased cost of maintenance energies such as heat and lights

    (Objective 3)

20. Which of the following has contributed to increases in health care costs?

    a. Increases in wages of health care workers

    b. Increases in physicians' charges

    c. The cost of new technology

    d. All of the above

    (Objective 3)

21. DRGs set a limit on which of the following?

    a. The amount of health care a person can receive

    b. The number of days of hospitalization allowed

    c. The reimbursement that the hospital will receive for care

    d. The number of diagnostic tests that may be performed

    (Objective 3)

22. What is a prospective payment system?

    a. One in which the hospital receives payment before the service is provided

    b. One in which the patient pays in advance for services needed

    c. One in which the hospital is paid a monthly sum by an insurance company for providing services at a special rate

    d. One in which the reimbursement amount for care is set ahead of time

    (Objective 3)

23. Which segment of our society has shown the greatest cost increases in the last 15 years?

    a. Food

    b. Housing

    c. Transportation

    d. Health care

    (Objective 3)

24. To assist in containing the cost of health care, the federal government has subsidized the creation of which of the following?

    a. Osteopathic hospitals

    b. Nontraditional approaches to health care

    c. Health maintenance organizations

    d. Emergency care centers

    (Objective 3)

25. What must a nurse do to create economic access?

    a. Gain skill in interviewing the client in regard to financial aspects of health care

    b. Learn how to correctly bill insurance carriers

    c. Lobby for universal health care coverage

    d. Relinquish high salary expectations

    (Objective 4)

26. What area has the most problems with geographic access to health care?

    a. Rural areas

    b. Suburban areas

    c. Urban areas

    d. Not identifiable

    (Objective 4)

27. An individual whose family is southeast Asian avoids going to health care providers because he feels people do not listen to his concerns. What problem does this individual have?

    a. Lack of cultural access to health care

    b. Deficit in acculturation to the American health care system

    c. Ineffective coping

    d. Impaired health seeking behavior

    (Objective 4)

28. Which of the following does NOT categorize access to health care services?

    a. Cultural access

    b. Economic access

    c. Personal access

    d. Geographic access

    (Objective 4)

29. What agency is primarily concerned with setting hospital standards?

    a. National League for Nursing

    b. Department of Health and Human Services

    c. State rate commission

    d. Joint Commission on Accreditation of Healthcare Organizations

    (Objective 5)

30. What agency is primarily concerned with evaluating and accrediting home health agencies?

    a. National League for Nursing

    b. Department of Education

    c. Community Health Accreditation Program

    d. Joint Commission on Accreditation of Healthcare Organizations

    (Objective 5)

31. What agency is primarily concerned with evaluating and accrediting health maintenance organizations?

    a. National League for Nursing

    b. National Committee for Quality Assurance

    c. Community Health Accreditation Program

    d. Joint Commission on Accreditation of Healthcare Organizations

    (Objective 5)

32. What agency or organization set the first standards requiring the evaluation of health care services?

    a. Medicare

    b. JCAHO

    c. CHAP

    d. NCQA

    (Objective 5)

33. PROs are charged with evaluating which of the following?

    a. Medical care

    b. Nursing care

    c. All aspects of the health care system

    d. Home care services

    (Objective 5)

34. What factor contributes most heavily to increasing power for nurses in the health care system?

    a. Nurses are seen in positive light by patients.

    b. Nurses have college education.

    c. Nurses are the largest single group of health care providers.

    d. Nurses are getting involved in political processes.

    (Objective 6)

35. Which group of health care providers has traditionally had the most power in health care?

    a. Physicians

    b. Nurses

    c. Hospital administrators

    d. Allied health professionals

    (Objective 6)

36. What is the most effective action a nurse could take to increase nurse power in a health care organization?

a. Nothing would change this situation.

b. Demand access to decision making.

c. Join with other nurses in seeking a more effective role.

d. Ask physicians to support more nursing power.

(Objective 6)

37. Government agencies possess what kind of power in health care?

    a. Charismatic power

    b. Positional power

    c. Regulatory power

    d. Persuasive power

    (Objective 6)

38. Who holds financial power in health care?

    a. Consumer

    b. Provider

    c. Third-party payer

    d. Accrediting agency

    (Objective 6)

39. Why are key indicators used in evaluating the health care system?

    a. They are the most important aspects of health care.

    b. They represent specific, measurable aspects of health care that can be used to evaluate the whole system.

    c. They are factors for which statistics are available.

    d. They are an exhaustive list of all the health care services that need to be evaluated.

    (Objective 7)

40. Which of the following describes the current status of health care reform?

    a. It is being considered by the federal government at this time.

b. It is moving to the state level of decision making.

c. It is part of the newly passed OBRA legislation.

d. It is no longer under consideration.

(Objective 7)

41. Health care cost increases are which of the following?

    a. A concern in countries that have socialized medicine also

    b. Unique to the United States

    c. Primarily a concern of Canada and the United States

    d. Not a major concern anywhere there is adequate care available

    (Objective 7)

42. What are nursing's major concerns for the future of health care?

    a. Maintaining an adequate supply of providers and providing adequate salaries for health care workers

    b. Supporting effective and strong regulations to maintain the current status

    c. Whether nursing's concerns for caring and individualization can be maintained in the face of cost containment

    d. How we will finance the newly legislated health care reforms

    (Objective 7)

## GAMING IN THE CLASSROOM

*Instructions: This game involves selecting teams and a host. The teams compete against one another for points. Each game has several subject categories. After teams are determined, a team is chosen to go first and selects a category. The host then poses the answer and the team provides the correct question for that answer. Each question can be awarded the same number of points or more difficult questions may be given heavier point values. (The instructor might determine which questions are more difficult based on the content emphasized in class.) Points are awarded to the team that is the first to signal and give a correct question. If that team is incorrect, the other team may attempt to provide the correct question and receive the points. The length of time allowed for response can be determined by the class or by the instructor. The team with the most points at the end of the game is declared the winner. Teams may be composed of individual students or groups of students. Teams may determine their answers as a team or may take turns answering as individuals.*

## Categories

A. Mechanisms for Funding Health Care

B. Federal Government Programs in Health Care

C. Cost Containment Strategies in Health Care

D. Access to Health Care

E. Power in Health Care

## Answers and Questions

### Category A

A: PPO.

Q: What is the designation given to a health care provider that contracts with an insurance company to provide services at a set, usually lower, price?

A: Capitation.

Q: What is the mechanism of payment in which a set fee is paid to the provider for each person enrolled regardless of amount of services used?

A: HMO.

Q: What is an organization that focuses on preventive care as a way of managing costs of health care?

A: Fee-for-service payment.

Q: What is the payment mechanism in which the more the services used the higher the fees that are paid?

A: Shared risk.

Q: What is the basic principle behind health insurance?

### Category B

A: Medicare.

Q: What is the federal program for funding health care for those on Social Security?

A: Charitable care.

Q: What were hospitals required to provide in order to receive federal funds for building?

A: Medicaid.

Q: What is the federal program administered through states that provides health care for the indigent?

A: CHAMPUS.

Q: What is the federal program to provide health care in the private sector for the military and dependents?

A: HCFA.

Q: What is the federal agency that manages the financial aspect of Medicare and Medicaid?

A: DRG.

Q: What is a payment category that Medicare has used to limit costs?

### Category C

A: Capitation.

Q: What mechanism limits costs by paying only a fixed amount per person enrolled regardless of services used?

A: Outliner.

Q: What is the term that indicates a person's hospital stay was significantly longer than average and, therefore, will receive additional reimbursement?

A: Comorbidity.

Q: What is the term for the presence of a second illness or complication that will result in additional reimbursement?

A: Restructuring.

Q: What is a reorganization of an agency called?

A: Prospective payment.

Q: What is the term for a predetermined payment for an illness or condition?

## Category D

A: Lack of translators.

Q: What is a cause of poor cultural access to health care?

A: Living in an economically depressed area.

Q: What is a cause of poor geographic access to health care?

A: Working for an employer that does not provide health insurance.

Q: What is a cause of poor economic access to health care?

A: Lack of responsiveness to religious beliefs.

Q: What is a cause of poor cultural access to health care?

A: Loans that can be repaid through working in an underserved area.

Q: What is a federal government program to increase geographic access to health care?

## Category E

A: Regulatory power.

Q: What type of power is controlled by governmental agencies?

A: Financial power.

Q: What type of power is controlled by third-party payers?

A: Connectional or collaborative power.

Q: What type of power is most available to nurses?

A: Physicians.

Q: What group of health care providers was most powerful in the past?

A: Limitations on physician power.

Q: What is an aspect of most health reform legislation?

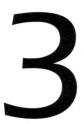

# 3

# The Political Process and the Nursing Profession

## PURPOSE

This chapter explores both the overall political process in which nurses may be engaged and the specific organizations that enter into this process. Within this chapter we provide the basis for understanding the political process and how it applies to health care. The role of the individual in the political process is emphasized, and specific information is presented on how the individual can participate and influence outcomes. The major federal legislation that has affected nursing in the past and current legislative concerns are presented. Common state and local political concerns are outlined. Organizations also have their own internal political processes; therefore, an understanding of the political process is relevant to members of an organization.

Many organizations are related to the nursing profession. These organizations affect the profession and can provide support to the individual nurse in numerous ways. The discussion of organizations in this chapter is directed toward helping the student understand these organizations, their purposes and activities, and how they relate to one another. The value of organizations for strengthening nursing's voice is emphasized. This information will provide direction as the student decides which organizations to join as a practicing nurse.

## OBJECTIVES

1. Explain the relevance of the political process to nursing.

2. Discuss seven ways you might influence the political process.

3. Outline the current U.S. federal governmental role in health care.

4. Explain common state legislative concerns.

5. Discuss common local political concerns.

6. Discuss the reasons for the existence of the large numbers of nursing organizations.

7. Discuss the major purpose of each specialized organization presented in the chapter.

8. Analyze the ways that nursing organizations seek to affect the health care delivery system and the political processes that control them.

9. Identify how politics is relevant to your participation in organizations.

## KEY TERMS

Allocation of resources
Americans with Disabilities Act (ADA)
Appropriations Act
Authorization Act
Conditions of participation
Department of Health and Human Services
Hatch Act
Lobbying
Minimum data set (MDS)
Nurse Practice Act
Occupational Safety and Health Act (OSHA)
Omnibus Budget Reconciliation Act (OBRA)
"Ontario" Plan
Political action committees (PACs)
Resident assessment protocols (RAPs)

## SITUATIONS TO FOSTER CRITICAL THINKING

1. Prepare an outline of how you would talk with other nurses to persuade them to register to vote and take an active part in working on a current legislative issue in your state. (Objective 1)

2. Examine the proposals currently being suggested to maintain the financial stability of the Medicare system. Identify the one you believe to be the best. Support your choice with rationale. (Objectives 2 and 3)

3. Identify a current health-related issue in your community. Present your own position on this issue with the rationale for your position. Determine where decisions will be made in regard to this issue. Outline the mechanisms you could use to influence decision making in regard to this issue. (Objectives 2 and 5)

4. Suppose that the Nurse Practice Act in your state will be subject to sunset review at the end of next year. What features of the current law are most important to you? What features would you like to change? What mechanisms are available to you to have input into this process? (Objectives 2 and 5)

5. The Public Health Department of your community is asking for public support for its outreach program for childhood immunization. What actions might you take to support this effort? (Objectives 2 and 5)

6. Review the nursing organizations listed in the Appendix. Choose three organizations and investigate their purposes, dues, structures, and benefits. Choose the one that you would join as a new graduate and provide rationale for your choice. (Objective 6)

7. You and another new graduate are discussing nursing organizations. She has asked whether you would join the specialty organization or the ANA. Identify your personal viewpoint and the rationale supporting your decision. (Objectives 7 and 9)

8. Some members of the nursing staff at the hospital where you work are putting together a proposal to support two nurses to attend a national convention of the ANA. Would you support this proposal? Outline the rationale underlying your position. Identify the strongest arguments in opposition to your position. (Objectives 7, 8, and 9)

9. A proposal is before a specialty organization to which you belong to join its certification program with the ANA Credentialing Center. Identify the benefits and the drawbacks for the specialty organization in losing its certification program. (Objectives 7 and 9)

10. Identify whether your nursing program is accredited by the NLN. What benefits are there in attending a nursing education program that is nationally accredited? Which of these benefits is of value to you and why? (Objectives 7 and 9)

11. Contact your state nurses association. Ask what legislative issues they are currently working on. Research these issues. Write a brief rationale of why the nurses association would be interested in this issue and what they might be doing to influence the political outcome. (Objective 8)

## DISCUSSION/ESSAY QUESTIONS

1. Identify one issue in which the political process is particularly relevant and explain why you think so. (Objective 1)

2. Define what is meant by the political process and explain how this might apply to an organization. (Objective 1)

3. What is lobbying and how might you participate in lobbying at the state level? (Objective 2)

4. What do you believe would have more effect on a federal legislator—a dozen signed form letters or one personally written letter? Explain your reasoning. (Objective 2)

5. Do you believe the Nurse Education Act should be funded by the federal government? Explain your position. (Objective 3)

6. Discuss the impact of two major provisions of the Nurse Education Act in the past. (Objective 3)

7. Who is covered by Medicare and how is Medicare financed? (Objective 3)

8. Discuss a recent change in the Medicare Act that has affected nursing practice. (Objective 3)

9. What governmental body administers the Medicare funds for families? On what is this based? How does this affect the delivery of nursing care services? (Objective 3)

10. Discuss the purpose of the OSHA and its impact on health care. (Objective 3)

11. What effect could the decreased federal funds for health care planning have on health care within a community? Explain your answer. (Objective 3)

12. One of the provisions of the Maternal Child Health Act was funding for research. How might this have an impact on nursing? (Objective 3)

13. What does catastrophic health coverage usually cover, and how might a decision of the state government to provide only this coverage for everyone affect the type of services that nurses would be providing? (Objective 4)

14. Where are the decisions about the content of the Nurse Practice Act made? (Objective 4)

15. When was the Nurse Practice Act in your state last changed? What effect might this have on the activities of your state nurses association? (Objective 4)

16. What is the major health responsibility of your local government? How might you affect the level of funding for this responsibility? (Objective 5)

17. What is a current major health problem in your community and how are nurses involved in solving it? (Objective 5)

18. Why are there so many different nursing organizations? (Objective 6)

19. What problems for nursing might the proliferation of organizations cause? (Objective 6)

20. What is the major function of the Board of Directors of the ANA? (Objective 7)

21. What is the role of the ANA in relationship to actions of the federal government? (Objective 7)

22. What services does the ANA provide that benefit the individual members? (Objective 7)

23. Outline the major areas that the NSNA addresses. (Objective 7)

24. What is the general purpose of the NLN? (Objective 7)

25. Give your views on why the NLN allows nonnurses as members. What benefits and what problems does this create for the organization? (Objective 8)

26. If two different scopes of practice for associate degree and baccalaureate nursing preparation become a standard, what do you believe the membership requirements for the ANA should be, and why? (Objective 8)

27. What is the role of the NLN in relationship to community health agencies? (Objective 8)

28. What is the NLN accreditation? Do you believe it is of value to a nursing program? Explain your answer. (Objective 8)

29. If you wish to change the policy of the American Nurses Credentialing Center regarding the BSN as a requirement for certification in a specialty, how would you do this? (Objective 9)

30. If you would like the nurses association in your state to support a legislative issue of interest to you, what should be your first action? (Objective 9)

31. You have decided to seek election as a member of the board of directors of your state nurses association. How will you use your understanding of the political process? (Objective 9)

32. You are unhappy with the public positions being taken by your state nurses association. How could you begin to affect those positions? (Objective 9)

33. You have determined that the current treasurer of your local specialty organization has not been keeping members informed. You note that a candidate for the position has taken this as a major goal. How would you use your knowledge of the political process to help this candidate be elected? (Objective 9)

## FILL IN THE BLANKS

*Instructions: Complete the following statements by filling in the blanks with the word or words that make the sentence complete and correct.*

1. Politics is the way in which people try to influence _____ _____ and the _____ of _____. (Objective 1)

2. Politics is found in both _____ and _____. (Objective 1)

3. The decision to join nursing organizations is usually a (an) _____ as well as a philosophical one. (Objective 1)

4. Historically, Florence Nightingale used political pressure to obtain _____ and _____. (Objective 1)

5. To influence the amount of money appropriated for the Nurse Education Act, you should contact your representative when the _____ _____ Act is being considered. (Objective 2)

6. The organization you would join to be a part of the ANA's political action efforts is _____. (Objective 2)

7. Three ways nurses can affect the political process are _____, _____ _____ _____, and _____ _____ _____. (Objective 2)

8. The changing role of _____ has been an important factor in the political activity of nurses. (Objective 2)

9. You can expect that the level of information available from television is primarily an _____. (Objective 2)

10. Issues of national interest are often highlighted in the ANA's official journal the _____ _____ _____ _____. (Objective 2)

11. Nursing organizations affect legislative issues by maintaining contact with _____ and _____ _____. (Objective 2)

12. Copies of federal legislation can be obtained from your _____ _____. (Objective 2)

13. When studying an issue, a key point is to identify _____ present in the source. (Objective 2)

14. The most fundamental way to participate in the political process in either an organization or the government is to _____. (Objective 2)

15. Legislators pay greater attention to a _____ letter than to a _____ letter. (Objective 2)

16. If you are employed by a governmental agency, you are more _____ in your political activity. (Objective 2)

17. The ANA has organized nurses to respond to political concerns through a group called _____. (Objective 2)

18. An organization that lobbies governmental agencies and the legislators is called a _____. (Objective 2)

19. The ANA political action committee is called _____. (Objective 2)

20. Employees of the federal government are limited in their political activity through the _____ Act. (Objective 2)

21. The Nurse Education Act provided funding for schools of nursing for _____ _____ and _____ _____. (Objective 3)

22. The two major sections of the Social Security Act that provide care for those over 65 and for dependent individuals are _____ and _____. (Objective 3)

23. The major purpose of OSHA is to _____ _____ _____. (Objective 3)

24. The major purpose of the Maternal-Child Health Act is to _____ _____ _____ _____ _____ _____ _____. (Objective 3)

25. Funds available from the federal government for any health care program must be approved in both an _____ and an _____ act. (Objective 3)

26. Nursing home regulations were contained in the federal legislation called _____. (Objective 3)

27. Issues relative to mental hospitals are usually decided at the _____ level. (Objective 4)

28. Scope of practice for nursing is determined in the _____ _____ Act. (Objective 4)

29. A new approach to licensing standards and scope of practice that identified 27 protected acts was initiated in _____. (Objective 4)

30. School health resources are usually determined at the _____ level. (Objective 5)

31. To influence the money allocated to a local immunization clinic, you would usually need to direct your efforts to the _____ government. (Objective 5)

32. Block grants consist of money from the federal government whose spending priorities are determined by the _____ government. (Objective 5)

33. Many of the new nursing organizations are organized around _____ practice. (Objective 6)

34. Many individuals choose to join specialty organizations because they provide _____ _____. (Objective 6)

35. The Constituent Assembly includes presidents and executive directors of _____ _____. (Objective 7)

36. "Facts About Nursing," a report of basic statistical information, is published by the _____. (Objective 7)

37. "Breakthrough into Nursing" is a project of the NSNA for the purpose of _____ _____ _____ _____. (Objective 7)

38. The prime purpose of the NLN is to _____ _____ _____ . (Objective 7)

39. In addition to nurses, _____ are eligible for membership in the NLN. (Objective 7)

40. The organization that provides for accreditation of nursing programs is the _____. (Objective 7)

41. The organization that provides for accreditation of agencies offering home health service is the _____. (Objective 7)

42. Is national accreditation of nursing programs voluntary or required? _____ (Objective 7)

43. The organization that recognizes individual nurses who have demonstrated outstanding scholarship and leadership for the profession is the _____ _____ _____ . (Objective 7)

44. The letters FAAN stand for _____ _____ _____ _____. (Objective 7)

45. The organization formed by the ANA as a political action arm is _____. (Objective 8)

46. The American Nurses Association tries to affect political outcomes through the _____. (Objective 8)

47. The _____ _____ _____ is most likely to support your interest in collective bargaining. (Objective 9)

48. You would join _____ to lobby for increased federal health care funding. (Objective 9)

# TRUE-FALSE QUESTIONS

*Instructions: Mark the following statements "T" if true or "F" if false. If using a scoring card, mark "A" if true or "B" if false.*

_____ 1. The political process consists only of what is done to influence the action of governmental bodies. (Objective 1)

_____ 2. The political process is a method of influencing decision making and the allocation of resources. (Objective 1)

_____ 3. The political process is not relevant to nurses. (Objective 1)

_____ 4. Decisions are made through the political process. (Objective 1)

_____ 5. Nurses working for a governmental agency may be prohibited from direct lobbying for funds. (Objective 2)

_____ 6. Lobbying is any communication with a government official. (Objective 2)

_____ 7. When you telephone a legislator, it is preferable to insist that you speak with that individual in person to ensure that your message is communicated. (Objective 2)

_____ 8. The federal government has input into health care only for those receiving Medicare and Medicaid funds. (Objective 3)

_____ 9. The original Nurse Training Act was passed in 1980. (Objective 3)

_____ 10. The Nurse Education (Training) Act has consistently been supported by the presidents of the United States throughout its existence. (Objective 3)

_____ 11. Because there is a shortage of nurses, the Nurse Education Act has been greatly expanded since 1990. (Objective 3)

_____ 12. Medicare serves only those who are 65 years of age and older. (Objective 3)

_____ 13. Support for renal dialysis is included in Medicare. (Objective 3)

_____ 14. Medicare provisions vary from state to state. (Objectives 3 and 5)

_____ 15. Hospitals are required to have a utilization and quality control review program. (Objective 3)

_____ 16. OSHA covers nurses in regard to exposure to toxic chemotherapeutic drugs. (Objective 3)

_____ 17. Most industrialized countries have systems for funding health care that are similar to those in the United States. (Objective 3)

_____ 18. Currently, federal assistance is available for those who do not have private health insurance. (Objective 3)

_____ 19. Budgets for institutions for the retarded and the mentally ill are usually determined at the state level. (Objective 4)

_____ 20. Nurse practice acts are state-level legislation. (Objective 4)

_____ 21. All states routinely reopen professional practice acts to determine whether they need to be changed. (Objective 4)

_____ 22. To influence money spent on an immunization project in your community, you would need to look to federal policies. (Objective 5)

_____ 23. The local health department is responsible for approving hospitals. (Objective 5)

_____ 24. Different nursing organizations have been formed to meet different needs identified in the profession. (Objective 6)

_____ 25. The House of Delegates of the ANA sets policy for the organization. (Objective 7)

_____ 26. The Board of Directors of the ANA sets policy for the organization. (Objective 7)

_____ 27. The ANA accredits schools of nursing. (Objective 7)

_____ 28. The ANA financially supports the NSNA. (Objective 7)

_____ 29. The ANA speaks for the profession of nursing to the general public. (Objective 7)

_____ 30. The NSNA is supporting the recruitment and retention of minorities in the field of nursing. (Objective 7)

_____ 31. The NSNA is a completely independent organization. (Objective 7)

_____ 32. The NLN promotes quality nursing care in all settings. (Objective 7)

_____ 33. Both organizations and individuals may join the NLN. (Objective 7)

_____ 34. Individual nurses may join the ANA directly. (Objective 7)

_____ 35. The NLN provides national accreditation for schools of nursing. (Objective 7)

_____ 36. The NLN does not involve itself in politics. (Objective 7)

_____ 37. National accreditation is required for graduates of a program to receive interstate endorsement of their licenses. (Objective 7)

_____ 38. Most specialty organizations provide continuing education for their members. (Objective 7)

_____ 39. FAAN stands for Fellow of the American Academy of Nursing. (Objective 7)

_____ 40. The American Nurses Foundation supports research in nursing. (Objective 7)

_____ 41. The National Council of State Boards of Nursing sets licensing requirements. (Objective 7)

_____ 42. Nursing organizations have separate but related entities that lobby on issues relevant to nursing. (Objective 8)

_____ 43. The ANA has lobbied in favor of expansion of the Nurse Education Act. (Objective 8)

_____ 44. The Tri-Council avoids speaking on issues that might be controversial within the nursing community. (Objective 8)

_____ 45. Running for an office in an organization is considered part of the political process of that organization. (Objective 9)

_____ 46. The techniques of lobbying for a position you favor can be used in a nursing organization. (Objective 9)

## MATCHING QUESTIONS

*Instructions: Match the numbered items with the most appropriate lettered items.*

### Group A (Objective 2)

_____ 1. Lobbying

_____ 2. Voting

_____ 3. Letter writing

_____ 4. E-mail

   a. Seeking to affect the decision of a legislator.

   b. A method of providing immediate input to a legislator.

   c. A personally developed one is more effective than a form.

   d. The most fundamental right of a citizen.

## Group B (Objective 3)

_____  1. O S & H Act

_____  2. Social Security Act

_____  3. Maternal-Child Act

_____  4. OBRA '87

a. Act that provides for Medicaid.

b. Act that provided nursing home regulations.

c. Act that included nutrition programs.

d. Act that mandated the use of "universal precautions" in health care.

## Group C (Objective 7)

_____  1. NSNA

_____  2. NLN

_____  3. ANA

_____  4. NCSBN

a. Organization that has both nurses and consumers as members.

b. Organization for students in programs leading to registered nurse licensure or higher nursing degrees.

c. Organization of state boards of nursing.

d. National professional organization with membership made up of state nurses associations.

## Group D (Objective 8)

_____  1. NLN

_____  2. ANA-PAC

_____  3. Tri-Council

_____  4. State nurses association

a. Organization that actively supports candidates for federal legislative offices.

b. Organization that provides expert testimony on health care issues for federal agencies and legislators.

c. Organization that works to achieve changes in the Nurse Practice Act that support nursing autonomy.

d. Organization that provides statistical information on nursing education.

## Group E (Objective 7)

_____  1. American Academy of Nursing

_____  2. Sigma Theta Tau

_____  3. Midwest Alliance in Nursing

_____  4. Nurses' House, Inc.

a. Organization of colleges and universities providing nursing education.

b. Organization providing financial assistance for nurses in need.

c. Organization of nurses with baccalaureate or higher degrees who have shown leadership and scholarship in nursing.

d. Organization of individuals who have made significant contributions to the field of nursing.

## MULTIPLE-CHOICE QUESTIONS

_Instructions: Choose the one best answer for each question._

1. What is one of the reasons the political process is relevant to nurses?

a. 35% of the U.S. population are nurses.

b. Many questions regarding health care are answered through legislation.

c. Nurses are required to report their voting activity.

d. Many nurses serve in state and national legislative positions.

(Objective 1)

2. Why is the political process relevant to nurses?

   a. One's practice as a nurse is controlled by a wide variety of governmental decisions.

   b. Many decisions are made within the various nurses' organizations.

   c. Health care is costly.

   d. Nurses may be drafted in case of war.

   (Objective 1)

3. What is one of the major concerns with regard to political issues as they are related to nursing?

   a. The lack of knowledge on the part of many nurses about the political process

   b. The lack of concern shown by nurses over broad health care issues

   c. The inability of nurses to get political attention

   d. The fact that so few voters are nurses

   (Objective 1)

4. Which of the following sources of information about political issues is most likely to be partisan toward a specific political party?

   a. A senator's newsletter

   b. The daily paper

   c. The Federal Registry

   d. A news magazine

   (Objective 2)

5. Which one of the following usually receives the least attention from a legislator?

   a. Mailgrams

   b. Personal letters

   c. Form letters

d. Telegrams

(Objective 2)

6. Which of the following results in the most immediate communication of your views to a legislator?

   a. Personal letter

   b. Mailgram

   c. Telephone call

   d. Express mail

   (Objective 2)

7. Which of the following is most critical for you to do to shape the political process?

   a. Be informed

   b. Influence others

   c. Run for office

   d. Write to your senator

   (Objective 2)

8. What is the federal agency concerned with planning for the organizations and personnel to provide health care in the community?

   a. National Institutes of Health

   b. Food and Drug Administration

   c. Office of Human Development Services

   d. Health Resources Administration

   (Objective 3)

9. The cabinet department originally identified as the Department of Health, Education, and Welfare is now known as which of the following?

   a. Office of Human Development

   b. United States Public Health Service

   c. Centers for Disease Control and Prevention

   d. Department of Health and Human Services

   (Objective 3)

10. The Public Health Service and the Food and Drug Administration are located in which cabinet department?

    a. Health and Human Services

    b. Interior

    c. Health Finance

    d. National Institutes of Health

    (Objective 3)

11. Which of the following is an outcome of the Nurse Education Act?

    a. It provided money for the construction of schools of nursing.

    b. It created an Institute of Nursing in Washington, DC.

    c. It funded the position of Chief Nurse of the United States Public Health Service.

    d. It established criteria for being a certified nursing assistant.

    (Objective 3)

12. Which federal act provided funds for nursing education?

    a. Social Security Act

    b. Comprehensive Health Planning Act

    c. Taft-Hartley Act

    d. Nurse Education (Training) Act

    (Objective 3)

13. Which of the following is one of the effects of the changes in the Nurse Education (Training) Act over the last 5 years?

    a. Increased financial aid for nursing students

    b. Decreased financial aid for nursing students

    c. Increased funding for construction of schools of nursing

    d. The channeling of funding away from advanced practice and research and toward basic educational programs

    (Objective 3)

14. In 1965, the Social Security Act was amended through Title VIII of the act, which was termed which of the following?

    a. Medicare

    b. Maternal-Child Health Act

    c. Health Planning and Utilization Act

    d. Medicaid

    (Objective 3)

15. The amount of money available under any federal legislative act depends on which of the following?

    a. The appropriated amount only

    b. The authorized amount only

    c. The agency's spending decisions

    d. All of the above

    (Objective 3)

16. What is the act that governs working conditions for nurses handling toxic chemotherapeutic agents?

    a. Maternal-Child Health Act

    b. OSHA

    C. Professional Standards Review Act

    d. Health Planning and Resources Development Act

    (Objective 3)

17. To affect the funding of health care for the state prison system, one would need to lobby which of the following?

    a. Department of Health and Human Services

    b. Congressional representative for one's district

c. Prison administrative officials

d. Budget committee for one's state legislature

(Objective 4)

18. Which level of government determines whether nurse practitioners are allowed to practice?

a. Federal level

b. State level

c. Local level

d. All of the above

(Objective 4)

19. To affect funding for the local health department, one would need to lobby which of the following?

a. United States Public Health Service

b. Congressional representative for one's district

c. Administrative officials of the public health department

d. County/city council

(Objective 5)

20. Health regulations for restaurants are usually regulated by which of the following?

a. Federal government

b. State government

c. Local government

d. None of the above

(Objective 5)

21. Which level of government usually supports school nurse funding?

a. Federal government

b. State government

c. Local government

d. None of the above

(Objective 5)

22. Which of the following is a serious concern raised by the existence of so many organizations in the field of nursing?

a. The restrictions on membership

b. The overlapping of function and interrelationships

c. Which one is the best organization

d. Which one is government approved

(Objective 6)

23. When nurses are deciding whether to join several nursing organizations, what is a major barrier?

a. Differences in basic philosophy between organizations

b. Cost of membership

c. Exclusionary policies of most nursing organizations

d. Time it takes to be a member

(Objective 6)

24. Which of the following is the major nursing organization that started with a meeting of nursing leaders at the World's Fair in Chicago in 1890?

a. NLN

b. Black Nurses Association

c. ANA

d. American College of Nurse Midwives

(Objective 7)

25. Which nursing organization has as one of its major concerns the economic welfare of nurses?

a. NLN

b. AWHONN

c. Association of Operating Room Nurses

d. ANA

(Objective 7)

26. Which of the following describes the NSNA?

    a. A branch of the ANA

    b. A branch of the NLN

    c. Supported by the American Hospital Association

    d. A fully independent organization

    (Objective 7)

27. The NLN supports quality nursing care through which of the following?

    a. Assisting nurses who are striving for better economic conditions

    b. Accrediting home health care agencies

    c. Giving scholarships to outstanding students in nursing

    d. Providing grants for nursing research

    (Objective 7)

28. Which nursing organization limits its membership to registered nurses?

    a. NLN

    b. American Public Health Association

    c. American Infection Control Association

    d. ANA

    (Objective 7)

29. Which nursing organization accredits nursing education programs?

    a. NLN

    b. NSNA

    c. ANA

    d. American Academy of Nursing

    (Objective 7)

30. What is the purpose of accreditation?

    a. Facilitate interstate movement of nurses

    b. Assist with licensure

    c. Support excellence in curriculum

    d. Help faculty know what should be taught

    (Objective 7)

31. In which nursing organization are new members elected by those currently in the organization?

    a. NLN

    b. American Academy of Nursing

    c. ANA

    d. American College of Nurse Midwives

    (Objective 7)

32. Which nursing organization meets once every 4 years?

    a. International Council of Nurses

    b. National Nursing Ethics Organization

    c. Federation of Nurse Practitioners

    d. ANA

    (Objective 7)

33. The delegates to the convention of the ANA are responsible for which of the following?

    a. Confirming all appointments to offices

    b. Determining the methods to be used to achieve goals

    c. Establishing the budget for the ANA

    d. Making policies to guide the organization

    (Objective 7)

34. The Board of Directors of the ANA is responsible for which of the following?

    a. Electing all officers

    b. Making policies

    c. Hiring the executive director

    d. Selecting representatives for the Constituent Assembly

    (Objective 7)

35. Which organization developed the Student Bill of Rights for nursing?

   a. ANA

   b. National Council of State Boards

   c. NLN

   d. NSNA

   (Objective 7)

36. Which of the following organizations is focused on nursing research?

   a. ANA

   b. American Nurses Foundation

   c. NLN

   d. NSNA

   (Objective 7)

## GAMING IN THE CLASSROOM

*Instructions: This game involves selecting teams and a host. The teams compete against one another for points. Each game has several subject categories. After teams are determined, a team is chosen to go first and selects a category. The host then poses the answer and the team provides the correct question for that answer. Each question can be awarded the same number of points or more difficult questions may be given heavier point values. (The instructor might determine which questions are more difficult based on the content emphasized in class.) Points are awarded to the team that is the first to signal and give a correct question. If that team is incorrect, the other team may attempt to provide the correct question and receive the points. The length of time allowed for response can be determined by the class or by the instructor. The team with the most points at the end of the game is declared the winner. Teams may be composed of individual students or groups of students. Teams may determine their answers as a team or may take turns answering as individuals.*

## Categories

A. Sources of Information about Political Issues

B. Influencing the Political Process

C. Federal Legislation Related to Health Care

D. State Government and Health Care

E. Purposes of Nursing Organizations

## Answers and Questions

### Category A

A: Bias.

Q: What should you examine sources of information for?

A: Common Cause.

Q: What is a consumer group that will provide information about political issues?

A: League of Women Voters.

Q: What is a nonpartisan group that will provide information about political issues?

A: Young Democrats and Young Republicans.

Q: What are politically partisan groups that will provide information about political issues?

A: Professional journals.

Q: What are sources of information about health-related political issues?

### Category B

A: Form letters.

Q: What is the least effective way to communicate with your legislator?

A: Personal letters.

Q: What is the communication with legislators that has the greatest impact?

A: The Honorable.

Q: What is the correct title for addressing a federal legislator?

A: Hatch Act.

Q: What federal act regulates political activity of government employees?

## Category C

A: Americans with Disabilities Act.

Q: What federal legislation requires access for those with disabilities?

A: Maternal-Child Act.

Q: What federal legislation has provided special help for women and children?

A: Social Security Act.

Q: What federal legislation provides for Medicare?

A: OBRA '97.

Q: What federal legislation provides for nursing home regulation?

A: OSHA.

Q: What federal legislation provides for workplace health and safety regulations?

## Category D

A: Public health department.

Q: What state agency establishes regulations for food handling?

A: Mental hospitals.

Q: What chronic care hospitals are usually supported by the state?

A: Nurse practice acts.

Q: What legislation does the state use to regulate nursing practice?

A: "Ontario" plan.

Q: What is the new approach to health professional licensing being considered by some states?

A: Professional licensing laws need more flexibility.

Q: What is a recommendation by the Pew Commission in regard to state health professional licensing?

## Category E

A: ANA.

Q: What nursing organization is formed by and for registered nurses?

A: NLN.

Q: What nursing organization has a major focus on nursing education?

A: AWHONN.

Q: Which nursing organization has a special focus on women's health, obstetrical, and neonatal nursing?

A: Sigma Theta Tau.

Q: Which international nursing organization was formed to honor scholarship and leadership in nursing?

A: NCSBN.

Q: Which nursing organization provides a forum for state boards of nursing to work together?

# 4

# Exploring Nursing's Origins

## PURPOSE

Chapter 4 explores the origin of nursing. It reviews the history of health care in early cultures and identifies any role that nursing may have had in those societies. The historical image of nursing is scrutinized followed by a discussion of the "Dark Ages of Nursing." The life of Florence Nightingale is discussed briefly, emphasizing the influence she had on the development of nursing as a profession. The impact of the Civil War on the development of the nursing profession is explored, and early nursing schools in the United States are described. The chapter concludes with a discussion of early nursing organizations and the history of the development of hospitals and nursing homes in the United States.

## OBJECTIVES

1. Describe the health care practices of early civilizations.

2. Analyze how each of the three historical images of the nurse has influenced the development of nursing as a profession.

3. Explain the significance of the "Dark Ages of Nursing" to the development of the nursing profession.

4. Discuss the contribution of Florence Nightingale to nursing and its development.

5. Explain the impact of the Civil War on the development of nursing in the United States.

6. Describe the early development of nursing schools in the United States.

7. Delineate the characteristics of early nursing programs.

8. Identify the first organizations created by and for nurses and discuss the purpose of each.

9. Discuss the history of hospitals and long-term care facilities in the United States.

10. Identify the factors that influenced the development of health care facilities and explain why each was important.

## KEY TERMS

Almshouse
Ancient cultures
Civil War
"Dark Ages of Nursing"
Flexner Report
Florence Nightingale
Folk image of nursing

Hospitals
Long-term care facilities
Nursing organizations
Pesthouse
Religious image of nursing
Servant image of nursing
"Uncommon women"

## SITUATIONS TO FOSTER CRITICAL THINKING

1. Review the health practices of early civilizations. Select one culture that you would like to visit if that were possible and identify why you chose that society. What questions would you want to ask about health care delivery in that culture? What would you want to observe? What relationships to today's health care practices could you identify? (Objective 1)

2. Of the three historical images of nursing discussed in your text, which do you believe had the strongest impact on nursing as a profession? Why do you believe this to be true? In what ways did it influence the development of nursing as a

profession? Was it a negative or positive impact? If it had been possible, how would you have changed the situation? (Objective 2)

3. Had you been in a position of power during the "Dark Ages of Nursing" what actions would you have taken regarding the practice of nursing? How would you have gone about making these changes? (Objective 3)

4. If you were able to sit down and have a cup of tea with Florence Nightingale, what would you want to ask her about nursing during the time she was alive? What would you want to share with her about nursing education today? How would you describe the role of the nurse in today's world to her? What questions do you think she would want to ask you? What comments do you think she would have regarding the role of the nurse today? (Objective 4)

5. Which events of the Civil War do you believe had the greatest impact on the development of nursing as a profession? Why do you believe this to be true? Is there a particular person associated with this event? What was that person's role? How would nursing be different today had this event not occurred? (Objective 5)

6. Imagine that you are a student in one of the early nursing programs. What do you see as the most striking difference between that program and the program in which you are currently enrolled? Are there any similarities? If so, what are they? What are your thoughts about the role of the nurse? (Objective 6)

7. What characteristics of the early nursing programs had the most impact on nursing as a profession? Why do you believe this to be true? Which characteristics of the early nursing programs had the least impact on nursing as a profession? Why do you believe this to be true? What changes would you have made in the way nursing education was initiated and

what impact do you believe that would have had on nursing education today? (Objective 7)

8. Imagine that you are attending the first meeting of the American Society of Superintendents of Training Schools in 1896. What do you think were the major agenda items at that meeting? Why have you selected those items? How do they relate to nursing today? How do you believe a president was selected for the group when there was no constitution or bylaws? (Objective 8)

9. Select one of the factors that affected the development of hospitals in the United States. Discuss how this factor was important and in what ways it influenced health care as we know it today. How might things be different if that force had been absent? Is it still critical today? Why or why not? (Objective 9)

10. What events or factors played a critical role in the development of hospitals and long-term care facilities in the United States? Why were these events or factors important? What was the purpose of the early hospitals in the late 1700s and early 1800s? Why was this so? (Objective 10)

## DISCUSSION/ESSAY QUESTIONS

1. Describe the approach to medicine seen in five early cultures, identifying the unique practices of each culture. (Objective 1)

2. Which of the early cultures do you believe had the most advanced approach to medicine? Defend you answer. (Objective 1)

3. Discuss the reasons that nursing did not possess a more prominent position in the health care of early civilizations. (Objective 1)

4. Identify the three historical images of nursing and indicate which you think most influenced the development of nursing as a profession, giving rationale. (Objective 2)

5. Of the three historical images of nursing, which one do you think is most reflected in nursing today? Explain your answer. (Objective 2)

6. What role did the early Deaconesses, Widows, and Virgins play in the development of nursing as a profession? (Objective 2)

7. How has nursing been influenced by early religious movements? (Objective 2)

8. What events led to the "Dark Ages" in nursing? (Objective 3)

9. Who was Sairey Gamp and what type of role did she portray? (Objective 3)

10. Discuss the contributions Florence Nightingale made to the nursing profession. (Objective 4)

11. Identify the characteristics Florence Nightingale stated as important in a good nursing education program. (Objective 4)

12. How has nursing been influenced by military activities? (Objectives 1, 2, and 5)

13. List three ways in which the Civil War affected the development of nursing in the United States and give an explanation for each. (Objective 5)

14. Identify four persons from Civil War times who made significant contributions to the development of nursing and explain why you believe each is significant. (Objective 5)

15. Discuss the early development of nursing education programs in the United States. (Objective 6)

16. What would you identify as obstacles to the establishment of early schools of nursing in the United States? Why do you believe these were obstacles? (Objective 6)

17. Describe the characteristics of early nursing education programs in the United States. (Objective 7)

18. Outline a day in the life of a nursing student enrolled in one of the early nursing education programs. (Objective 7)

19. Which was the oldest nursing organization and when was it founded? (Objective 8)

20. What events came together and resulted in the formation of the first nursing organization? (Objective 8)

21. What was the purpose(s) of the first nursing organization? (Objective 8)

22. What nursing organizations were being formed in other countries at the time nursing organizations were starting in the United States? (Objective 8)

23. Discuss the development of the National League for Nursing. (Objective 8)

24. Where were the first hospitals founded in the United States? (Objective 9)

25. What was an almshouse and what was its purpose? (Objective 9)

26. What legislation preceded the founding of hospitals in the United States? (Objective 9)

27. Discuss the development of early hospitals and explain why they were located where they were. (Objective 9)

28. What is the history of long-term care facilities in the United States? (Objective 9)

29. List three factors that influenced the development of health care facilities and explain why each is important. (Objective 10)

30. Of the factors influencing the development of health care facilities, which one do you believe is most important? Why? (Objective 10)

# FILL IN THE BLANKS

*Instructions: Complete the following statements by filling in the blanks with the word or words that make the sentence complete and correct.*

1. In the ancient Egyptian culture, treating disease was considered the responsibility of _____. (Objective 1)

2. The oldest medical records so far discovered and deciphered are those from _____. (Objective 1)

3. The Babylonians believed illness to be the _____ ___ ____ and for _____ ___ _____. (Objective 1)

4. The Father of Medicine, Hippocrates, was born about 400 B.C. on the island of Cos in _____. (Objective 1)

5. The genius of the Romans found its best expression in the area of _____ _____. (Objective 1)

6. The religious philosophy of Buddhism was developed by _____ _____. (Objective 1)

7. The development of elaborate materia medica was of major significance in ancient _____. (Objective 1)

8. In early American culture, the _____ had hospices for the care of the ill, used minerals as drugs, used soporifics to decrease pain, and assisted women with childbirth. (Objective 1)

9. Three images that have been associated with the history of nursing include the _____ image, the _____ image, and the _____ image. (Objective 2)

10. One group of women of particular significance to the history of nursing were the _____ of the Eastern Christian Church. (Objective 2)

11. Because the Order of Widows and the Order of Virgins often visited the sick in their homes, they are sometimes recognized as the earliest organized group of ____ _____ _____. (Objective 2)

12. Three Roman "matrons" who are remembered in the history of nursing are _____, _____, and _____ _____. (Objective 2)

13. One of the earliest organizations for men in nursing is the _____ _____. (Objective 2)

14. An 11th century Muslim "Nightingale," who nursed during the time of the Prophet Mohammed, was _____ _____. (Objective 2)

15. One of the outcomes of the Reformation that significantly affected nursing was a _____ ____ ____ _____ ___ _____. (Objective 3)

16. The "Dark Ages" in nursing were precipitated by the _____ _____. (Objective 3)

17. A character from a book by Martin Chuzzlewit to whom we often attribute all the bad images of nursing during the "Dark Ages of Nursing" was _____ _____. (Objective 3)

18. During the early 1600s several nursing groups were organized in Europe; they included the ____ __ _____ __ ____, and __ _____ __ _____. (Objective 3)

19. The first hospital on the American continent was the _____ _____ _____ _____ in Mexico City. (Objectives 3 and 8)

20. The _____ _____, an order of teaching nuns, is credited with attempting to organize the first training for nurses on this continent. (Objective 3)

21. The individual who reformed the care of British soldiers wounded in the Crimean War was _____ _____. (Objective 4)

22. One of the major accomplishments of Florence Nightingale was the _____ ____ _____ _____ ____ _____. (Objective 4)

23. The ____ _____, a steamer converted into a floating hospital, is considered the first Navy hospital ship. (Objective 5)

24. The American Red Cross was founded by
    _____ _____. (Objective 5)

25. The first nursing program was established
    at the ___ ___ ____ __ _____ in
    1872. (Objective 6)

26. Initially, nursing education was largely
    an _____ and resulted in students
    providing much of the _____
    of hospitals. (Objective 6)

27. The earliest nursing textbook is reported-
    ly the _____ __ _____ __ _____ __
    _____ ___. (Objective 6)

28. The first nurses' meeting was held at the
    _____ ____ in _____ in 1893.
    (Objective 8)

29. The first hospital founded in the United
    States was started in _____ in
    _____. (Objective 9)

30. The first hospital in the United States was
    founded at the urging of _____
    _____. (Objective 9)

31. The early hospitals did not admit the
    mentally ill; one of the facilities to first
    offer this type of care was _____
    _____ _____ _____. (Objective 9)

32. A woman who crusaded against the cruel
    and inhumane treatment of patients in
    the early mental hospitals was _____
    _____. (Objective 9)

33. Major forces resulting in the develop-
    ment of hospitals included _____,
    _____, _____, and
    _____. (Objective 10)

34. The _____ _____ led to changes in
    the structure and content of curricula in
    medical schools. (Objective 10)

35. Almshouses and poorhouses were con-
    structed by the government in the 1800s
    to shelter the _____ _____.
    (Objective 9)

36. The first hospital insurance plan was ini-
    tiated at _____ _____ _____ in 1929 to
    serve the needs of schoolteachers in
    _____, _____. (Objective 10)

37. As a result of the ____ _____ ____ of
    1935, private nursing homes emerged
    during that decade. (Objectives 9 and 10)

38. During the time following World War II
    the _____ __ _____ was passed, which
    supported hospital construction.
    (Objectives 9 and 10)

39. Two of the purposes of the American
    Hospital Association, when it was found-
    ed in 1899, were to _____ and
    _____. (Objective 10)

40. For nursing homes to collect Medicare
    dollars, they must be _____ as
    _____ _____ _____. (Objective 10)

## TRUE-FALSE QUESTIONS

*Instructions: Mark the following statements
"T" if true or "F" if false. If using a scoring card,
mark "A" if true or "B" if false.*

_____ 1. The earliest medical records so far
    discovered and deciphered are those
    from Egypt, dating back as far as
    3000 B.C. (Objective 1)

_____ 2. The Mosaic Code emphasized the
    isolation of people with communi-
    cable diseases and differentiated
    clean from unclean. (Objective 1)

_____ 3. The early Babylonians are credited
    with developing beginning concepts
    related to the "germ theory" of dis-
    ease. (Objective 1)

_____ 4. The early Assyrians believed in
    Zoroaster, a prophet who wrote
    sacred books. (Objective 1)

_____ 5. The Father of Medicine, Hippocrates,
    was born about 400 B.C. on the
    island of Cos in Greece. (Objective 1)

_____ 6. Cleanliness was valued in the early
    Roman society. (Objective 1)

_____ 7. The citizens of early India had little understanding of disease prevention, hygiene, or sanitation. (Objective 1)

_____ 8. The philosophy of the yang and the yin was developed by the early Indian culture. (Objective 1)

_____ 9. Dissection was performed in China before 2000 B.C. (Objective 1)

_____ 10. Although ancient cultures developed medicine as a science and a profession they showed little evidence of establishing a foundation for nursing. (Objective 1)

_____ 11. Because nursing developed an image closely tied to religion and religious orders, strict discipline was expected. (Objective 2)

_____ 12. St. Marcella is often referred to as the first deaconess and the first visiting nurse. (Objective 2)

_____ 13. The Hospitallers of St. John was one of the orders to evolve from the Civil War. (Objective 2)

_____ 14. Continuity in the history of nursing began with Christianity. (Objective 2)

_____ 15. The military nursing orders were eliminated by the Crusades. (Objective 2)

_____ 16. A Muslim nurse, Rufaida Al-Asalmiya, provided care to members of the Muslim army during the holy war, and her efforts have been likened to those of Florence Nightingale. (Objective 2)

_____ 17. The image of nurses developed through the character of Sairey Gamp portrayed nursing in a very positive light. (Objective 3)

_____ 18. The Reformation led to the establishment of Catholic churches and hospitals throughout Europe. (Objective 3)

_____ 19. Florence Nightingale crusaded for and brought about great reform in nursing education. (Objective 4)

_____ 20. Florence Nightingale believed that an important aspect of nurses' work involved cleaning. (Objective 4)

_____ 21. Florence Nightingale was the first nursing supervisor of St. Elizabeth's Hospital in London. (Objective 4)

_____ 22. We honor the memory of Florence Nightingale through National Hospital Week, which occurs the week we celebrate the anniversary of her birth. (Objective 4)

_____ 23. At the time of the Civil War there were well-established MASH units and the beginning of an army nurse corps. (Objective 5)

_____ 24. The serious need for trained nurses, created by the Civil War, was undoubtedly a significant factor in the development of nursing in the United States. (Objective 5)

_____ 25. Sojourner Truth nursed Union soldiers, worked for improvement in sanitary facilities, and sought contributions of food and clothing for black volunteer regiments during the Civil War. (Objective 5)

_____ 26. Louisa May Alcott served as a volunteer nurse during the Civil War and from her experiences wrote *Hospital Sketches,* which depicted much of the suffering that occurred. (Objective 5)

_____ 27. After the Civil War, the American Medical Association fought the development of nursing education programs. (Objective 5 and 6)

_____ 28. The New England Hospital for Women and Children is often credited with being the first hospital to establish a formal one-year program to train nurses in 1872. (Objective 6)

_____ 29. Lavinia Dock is acknowledged as America's first trained nurse. (Objective 6)

_____ 30. The curricula of the early nursing schools were heavily standardized and all programs were accredited by the American Medical Association. (Objective 7)

_____ 31. Mills School of Nursing at Bellevue Hospital in New York was the first school established for male nurses that prepared them to give general patient care. (Objective 7)

_____ 32. Prior to 1901, there were five different journals published for nurses. (Objective 8)

_____ 33. In 1893, Florence Nightingale attended the first meeting of what would eventually become the American Nurses Association and gave an address. (Objective 8)

_____ 34. The first hospital founded in the United States was started in Philadelphia in 1751. (Objective 9)

_____ 35. Benjamin Franklin fought hospital development in the United States. (Objective 9)

_____ 36. The first nursing homes in the United States were established after the Social Security Act of 1935 was passed. (Objective 9)

_____ 37. The early hospitals included in their structure a section for the treatment of the mentally ill. (Objective 9)

_____ 38. A major impetus to the growth of hospitals in the United States was the development of professional nursing. (Objective 10)

_____ 39. The growth of the health insurance industry did little to foster the development of hospitals throughout the United States. (Objective 10)

_____ 40. The American Hospital Association was founded in 1899 as the Association of Hospital Superintendents with a membership of nine. (Objective 10)

# MATCHING QUESTIONS

_Instructions: Match the numbered items with the most appropriate lettered items._

## Group A (Objective 1)

_____ 1. Developed a pharmacopoeia classifying more than 700 drugs.

_____ 2. Developed the Mosaic Code, which included methods of disease prevention.

_____ 3. Developed the Code of Hammurabi, regarding payment of fees for care.

_____ 4. Had well-developed practices of hygiene and sanitation.

_____ 5. Their practice of surgery may have been the most highly developed of any ancient culture.

_____ 6. Health practices based on philosophy of yin and yang focused on prevention and good health.

a. Greece

b. India

c. Egypt

d. China

e. Palestine

f. Rome

## Group B (Objective 2)

_____ 1. A Roman woman of means who made her luxurious home into a monastery.

_____ 2. Assisted St. Jerome in the translation of the writings of the prophets.

_____ 3. Served as grand master of the Knights Hospitallers of St. John.

_____ 4. Often referred to as the first deaconess and first visiting nurse.

_____ 5. Cared for Muslim soldiers during the holy war.

   a. Phoebe

   b. Rufaida Al-Asalmiya

   c. Gerard

   d. St. Paula

   e. Marcella

## Group C (Objective 5)

_____ 1. Worked as a nurse/counselor for the Freedmen's Relief Association after the Civil War.

_____ 2. Was commissioned as Superintendent of Women Nurses for All Military Hospitals during the Civil War.

_____ 3. Challenged the work of lazy and corrupt medical officers during the Civil War.

_____ 4. An abolitionist sometimes called "Conductor of the Underground Railroad" who nursed soldiers during the Civil War.

_____ 5. A Civil War nurse who was instrumental in founding the American Red Cross in 1882.

_____ 6. Worked as a volunteer nurse in the Civil War after searching for a brother who had been wounded.

   a. Clara Barton

   b. Walt Whitman

   c. Sojourner Truth

   d. Dorothea Dix

   e. Harriet Ross Tubman

   f. Mary Ann Ball Bickerdyke

## Group D (Objective 9)

_____ 1. One of the first hospitals constructed that divided the facility into wards or pavilions, each one a separate building.

_____ 2. The first hospital in the United States.

_____ 3. The first hospital on the North American Continent.

_____ 4. One of the first mental hospitals in the United States.

_____ 5. Established primarily to prevent the spread of infectious diseases brought by sailors and immigrants.

   a. Friend's Hospital

   b. Hospital of the Immaculate Conception

   c. New York Hospital

   d. Massachusetts General Hospital

   e. Pennsylvania Hospital

## MULTIPLE-CHOICE QUESTIONS

*Instructions: Choose the one best answer for each question.*

1. Which of the following early cultures is credited with having the oldest medical records so far discovered?

   a. China

   b. Egypt

   c. India

   d. Persia

   (Objective 1)

2. Which of the following is an early culture that developed an organized method of disease prevention?

   a. Babylonia

   b. Egypt

c. India

d. Palestine

(Objective 1)

3. Which early culture developed an elaborate materia medica?

   a. Babylonians

   b. Brahmans

   c. Chinese

   d. Persians

   (Objective 1)

4. Which ancient culture is credited with the books of Ayur Veda that discussed children's diseases?

   a. India

   b. Palestine

   c. Persia

   d. Rome

   (Objective 1)

5. Which of the following images of nursing was inherited from the medieval period?

   a. The folk image

   b. The professional image

   c. The religious image

   d. The servant image

   (Objective 2)

6. Which of the following is one of the three historical images of the nurse identified by Uprichard?

   a. Angel of mercy

   b. Battle-axe

   c. Folk

   d. Handmaiden

   (Objective 2)

7. The early deaconesses sometimes are identified as the early counterpart of which branch of nursing today?

   a. Community health nurses

   b. Epidemiologists (disease control nurses)

   c. Nurse anesthetists

   d. Nurse practitioners

   (Objective 2)

8. Which image of the nurse was a product of the "Dark Ages of Nursing"?

   a. The folk image

   b. The professional image

   c. The religious image

   d. The servant image

   (Objective 2)

9. Which of the follow represents one of the earliest organizations for men in nursing?

   a. The Alexian Brothers

   b. The Knights Hospitallers of St. John

   c. The Knights of the Teutonic Order

   d. The Parabolani brotherhood

   (Objective 2)

10. Who was one of the early Roman matrons who significantly contributed to nursing by opening her home as a monastery for women?

    a. Anastasia

    b. Christina

    c. Marcella

    d. St. Maria

    (Objective 2)

11. When were the Order of Visitation of Mary, St. Vincent de Paul, and the Sisters of Charity established in Europe?

    a. 1500s

    b. 1600s

    c. 1700s

    d. 1800s

    (Objectives 2 and 3)

12. Which of the following nursing orders established a nursing order in the United States under the direction of Elizabeth Bayley Seton?

    a. Order of the Visitation of Mary

    b. Sisters of Charity

    c. Sisters of Providence

    d. St. Vincent de Paul

    (Objective 3)

13. Where was the first medical school on the North American continent founded?

    a. Mexico City

    b. New York City

    c. Philadelphia

    d. Toronto

    (Objective 3)

14. The effects of the Reformation during the 16th century created which of the following in nursing?

    a. The birth of modern nursing

    b. The "Dark Ages" in nursing

    c. The development of nursing schools

    d. The Renaissance

    (Objective 3)

15. How did the Reformation affect nursing?

    a. It changed the role of the Pope.

    b. It changed the role of women at that time.

    c. It encouraged people to be free thinkers.

    d. It enhanced the image of nursing at that time.

    (Objective 3)

16. Who is credited with establishing a training institute for deaconesses at Kaiserwerth in Germany?

    a. Elizabeth Fry

    b. Florence Nightingale

    c. Pastor Theodore Fliedner

    d. The Parabolani brotherhood

    (Objective 4)

17. Florence Nightingale cared for soldiers in which war?

    a. The Crimean War

    b. The Crusades

    c. The Revolutionary War

    d. The War of 1812

    (Objective 4)

18. Which represents one of Florence Nightingale's beliefs about nursing education?

    a. All instruction would be directed by physicians.

    b. Records would be kept on the students.

    c. The curriculum should include only theoretical teaching.

    d. The teachers should not receive remuneration for their services.

    (Objective 4)

19. In what way do we honor the memory of Florence Nightingale today?

    a. All Saints Day

    b. National Hospital Week

    c. National Teacher's Week

    d. Nurse Education Week

    (Objective 4)

20. Which was one of Florence Nightingale's major contributions to nursing?

    a. Bringing nurses to the war front

    b. Establishing a profession separate from medicine

    c. Establishing a registry for nurses

d. Establishing standards for schools of nursing

(Objective 4)

21. Who authored one of the first books on the organization of training schools of nursing?

a. Abby Howland Woolsey

b. Georgeanna Muirson Woolsey

c. Susie Taylor King

d. Walt Whitman

(Objectives 5 and 6)

22. Who was instrumental in founding the American Red Cross?

a. Abby Howland Woolsey

b. Clara Barton

c. Dorothea Dix

d. Mary Ann Ball Bickendyke

(Objective 5)

23. Which state was one of the first to recommend that institutions be formed to educate nurses?

a. Alabama

b. Delaware

c. Massachusetts

d. New York

(Objective 6)

24. Which is true of the early schools in the United States?

a. They had fairly standard curricula.

b. They were fashioned after the Nightingale model.

c. They were founded in colleges and universities.

d. They were well financed.

(Objective 7)

25. Who was the first black nurse to graduate from a nursing program in the United States?

a. Harriet Ross Tubman

b. Mary Eliza Mahoney

c. Sojourner Truth

d. Susie King Taylor

(Objective 7)

26. Which of the following was one of the reasons for the establishment of the early nursing programs?

a. Provide assistants to the physicians

b. Provide expanded roles in health care

c. Provide jobs for women

d. Provide a work force for the hospitals

(Objective 7)

27. Which of the following was identified as a problem as early as 1905?

a. Increase in acuity in hospitals

b. Lack of qualified nursing faculty

c. Proliferation of nursing programs

d. Shortage of nurses

(Objective 7)

28. Which of the following was the title of an early nursing textbook?

a. *Harmer and Henderson's Medical Surgical Nursing*

b. *Nursing: Its Principles and Practices for Hospital and Private Use*

c. *The Basic Facts about Nursing*

d. *The First Primer on Nursing*

(Objective 7)

29. The Nurses' Associated Alumnae of the United States and Canada was the forerunner of which current nursing association?

a. American Nurses Association

b. Association of Nurse Anesthetists

c. International Council of Nurses

d. National League for Nursing

(Objective 8)

30. When was the International Council of Nurses formed?

    a. 1750

    b. 1800

    c. 1899

    d. 1959

    (Objective 8)

31. Which of the following was one of the major purposes of the International Council of Nurses?

    a. To increase nurses' salaries around the world

    b. To enhance the image of nursing around the world

    c. To provide opportunities for nurses from all parts of the world to meet and discuss concerns

    d. To provide opportunities for nurses from all parts of the world to develop approaches to nursing research

    (Objective 8)

32. What was the name associated with early facilities built to isolate people with contagious diseases?

    a. Almshouses

    b. Asylums

    c. Convents

    d. Pesthouses

    (Objective 9)

33. Where was the first hospital in the United States founded?

    a. Detroit

b. Gettysburg

c. Hartford

d. Philadelphia

(Objective 9)

34. Who was the individual who campaigned vigorously for and brought much reform in the area of mental health treatment?

    a. Clara Barton

    b. Dorothea Dix

    c. Margaret Sanger

    d. Lillian Wald

    (Objective 9)

35. One of the early reports addressed changes in the structure and content of curricula in medical schools. What was it called?

    a. Brown Report

    b. Carnegie Study

    c. Flexner Report

    d. Institute of Medicine Study

    (Objective 9)

36. For whom was the first hospital insurance plan initiated?

    a. Automotive workers

    b. Nurses

    c. Physicians

    d. Teachers

    (Objective 9)

37. Which of the following health care plans is modeled after the plan originally established at Baylor University Hospital in 1929.

    a. Aetna

    b. Blue Cross

    c. HMOs

    d. Teamsters

    (Objective 9)

38. What federal legislation provided support for hospital construction?

    a. Hill-Burton Act

    b. Nurse Training Act

    c. Social Security Act of 1935

    d. Wagner Act

    (Objective 10)

39. What is required of nursing homes in order that they collect Medicare funds?

    a. That all care be provided by registered nurses

    b. That all patients have developed living wills

    c. That the facility have a 24-hour pharmacist on site

    d. That the facility be certified as a skilled nursing facility

    (Objective 10)

40. Which of the following was one of the purposes of the American Hospital Association when it was founded?

    a. Establish and maintain high standards of hospital service

    b. Influence legislation

    c. Provide communication among hospital administrators

    d. Recruit nurses

    (Objective 10)

## GAMING IN THE CLASSROOM

*Instructions: This game involves selecting teams and a host. The teams compete against one another for points. Each game has several subject categories. After teams are determined, a team is chosen to go first and selects a category. The host then poses the answer and the team provides the correct question for that answer. Each question*
can be awarded the same number of points or more difficult questions may be given heavier point values. (The instructor might determine which questions are more difficult based on the content emphasized in class.) Points are awarded to the team that is the first to signal and give a correct question. If that team is incorrect, the other team may attempt to provide the correct question and receive the points. The length of time allowed for response can be determined by the class or by the instructor. The team with the most points at the end of the game is declared the winner. Teams may be composed of individual students or groups of students. Teams may determine their answers as a team or may take turns answering as individuals.*

## Categories

A. Early Health Care Practices

B. Historical Nurses and Nursing

C. Florence Nightingale

D. Early Nursing Schools

E. Early Hospitals

## Answers and Questions

### Category A

A: An early culture skilled in wrapping and embalming the dead.

Q: What is Egypt?

A: Under the leadership of Moses, this country developed the Mosaic Code, which included an organized method of disease prevention.

Q: What is Palestine?

A: In Hebrew culture, these individuals taught that visiting the sick was a duty.

Q: Who were the early Jewish rabbis?

A: This early prophet, who wrote the sacred books of Persia, introduced the concept of two creators —one good and one evil.

Q: Who was Zoroaster?

A:  The country that was home to Hippocrates.

Q:  What is Greece?

## Category B

A:  Groups organized in early churches to care for the sick, poor, orphans, widows, and aged.

Q:  What are Orders?

A:  They are often considered the early counterparts of today's community health nurses.

Q:  Who were the early deaconesses?

A:  She worked as a scholar of Marcella and assisted St. Jerome in the translation of the writings of the prophets.

Q:  Who was St. Paula?

A:  A hospital established in Lyons in England in 542.

Q:  What is the Hotel Dieu?

A:  A Belgian secular order started in 1184.

Q:  What were the Beguines of Flanders?

A:  She built a hospice at Ostia to care for strangers.

Q:  Who was Fabiola?

## Category C

A:  At an institute in Kaiserwerth, Germany.

Q:  Where did Florence Nightingale study nursing?

A:  He was a friend of Florence Nightingale's and was instrumental in involving her in the care of Crimean War casualties.

Q:  Who was Sir Sidney Herbert?

A:  A nursing facility of which Florence Nightingale was superintendent.

Q:  What was the Establishment for Gentlewomen During Illness?

A:  An award given to Florence Nightingale in 1907 by the Queen of England.

Q:  What is the Order of Merit?

A:  A school of nursing in England financed by the Nightingale Trust Fund.

Q:  What is St. Thomas' Hospital in London?

## Category D

A:  A historical event in the United States that emphasized the need for trained nurses.

Q:  What was the Civil War?

A:  Credited with being the first hospital to establish a formal one-year program to train nurses.

Q:  What was the New England Hospital for Women and Children?

A:  The first nursing graduate in the United States.

Q:  Who was Melinda Ann (Linda) Richards?

A:  A characteristic of education typified by the early nursing programs.

Q:  What is an apprenticeship?

A:  Established as the first separate school to educate black nurses.

Q:  What was Spelman Seminary in Atlanta, Georgia?

## Category E

A:  The forerunner of hospitals in the United States.

Q:  What were almshouses?

A:  Services that were not provided in the early hospitals.

Q:  What was care for the mentally ill?

A:  Advances in medical science and medical technology.

Q:  What are two factors that served as major forces in the development of hospitals in the United States?

A:  An act resulting in the construction of hospitals throughout the United States.

Q:  What was the Hill-Burton Act?

A:  A term that encompasses a side spectrum of facilities that can range from special units in acute community hospitals to a campus of care retirement centers.

Q:  What are nursing homes today?

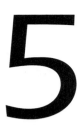

# Nursing as a Developing Profession

## PURPOSE

Chapter 5 discusses the development of nursing as a profession and makes distinctions between nursing and medicine. It outlines the characteristics of a profession described by social scientists and discusses the challenges offered to nursing with regard to these characteristics. The image of nursing today is reviewed, and how that image affects the profession is explored. Studies about nursing are described and their impact on the profession reviewed. The chapter concludes with a discussion of the traditions in nursing including pinning, caps, and uniforms.

## OBJECTIVES

**1.** Analyze the reasons the profession has had difficulty defining nursing.

**2.** Describe how nursing differs from medicine.

**3.** Formulate a personal definition of nursing and identify a theorist who defines nursing similarly.

**4.** Identify the seven characteristics that social scientists use to evaluate professions.

**5.** Discuss the application of these seven characteristics to nursing as a profession.

**6.** Compare and contrast the terms profession and professional.

**7.** Explain how the image others hold of nursing affects the profession and the role of the nurse.

**8.** Analyze areas of nursing about which studies have been conducted and discuss why each is important.

**9.** Describe some of the traditions in nursing and consider why they became traditions.

## KEY TERMS

Body of specialized knowledge

Code of ethics

Formal characteristics

Image

Institutions of higher education

Lifetime commitment

Medicine

Nursing

Occupation

Profession

Professional

Professional activity

Professional policy

Service to the public

Studies about nursing

Traditions

## SITUATIONS TO FOSTER CRITICAL THINKING

1. What are the factors in the development of nursing as a profession that have made it difficult to provide an exact definition of nursing? How might these factors have been changed? Do you believe it is a problem for the profession? Why or why not? Is it something about which we, as nurses, should be concerned? Why or why not? (Objective 1)

2. Explain the relationship you see between nursing and medicine? Why do differences exist? Are they significant? How could the differences affect the working relationships between members of the two professions? Does the history of gender differences play a role in the image we hold for each profession today? In what ways? (Objective 2)

3. Develop a definition of nursing that

reflects your beliefs about the role and responsibilities of today's nurse. Compare and contrast your definition with the definitions of three major nursing theorists. Defend concepts that you have included that differ from those of each theorist. Why did you choose to include those concepts in your definition of nursing? (Objective 3)

4. You are asked to do a presentation for a group of prenursing students on nursing as a profession. Using the characteristics typically associated with professions, what factors will you emphasize? Which factors will you omit? Why did you make those choices? Are there additional factors that you believe should be considered? Provide a rationale for all of your answers. (Objective 4)

5. Of the seven major characteristics of a profession that social scientists use to measure professions, which one do you believe is the most important? Why? Which do you believe is the least important? Why? What is the role of a code of ethics? Why do you believe this was included in the major characteristics of a profession? (Objective 5)

6. What are the factors that have created confusion about the use of the terms *profession* and *professional*? Do you think these factors are of any real importance? Why or why not? Do you believe such items as attitude, dress, conduct, and deportment should make a difference? Why or why not? (Objective 6)

7. Identify ways in which you believe that the image others have of nursing affects the profession. Do you believe that the majority of people view nurses and nursing positively? If you were to poll your nonnurse friends and colleagues regarding their perception of nurses and nursing, what do you believe they would tell you? Do you think those perceptions would change if your friends had a recent hospitalization? Why or why not? (Objective 7)

8. Identify at least three issues that you believe need to be studied with regard to nursing as it is currently being practiced. Provide a rationale for these studies. How will nursing benefit from the studies? Who should do the studies? What might be some of the outcomes? What might be the impact on health care reform? (Objective 8)

9. Take a position on one of the traditions in nursing. Develop a rationale for its continuance or demise. What will be the effect of either? On whom? Would it make any difference to nursing as a profession? Why or why not? (Objective 9)

## DISCUSSION/ESSAY QUESTIONS

1. What factors have hampered the profession in defining nursing? (Objective 1)

2. Do you believe nursing is both an art and a science? Why or why not? (Objective 1)

3. What do you believe are the major differences between the profession of nursing and the profession of medicine? (Objective 2)

4. Do you believe nursing is a part of the field of medicine? Why or why not? (Objective 2)

5. Which nursing theory does your personal definition of nursing most closely parallel and who was its author? (Objective 3)

6. From a personal perspective, defend or refute the statement, "A nurse, is a nurse, is a nurse." (Objective 3)

7. Should nursing be considered a profession or an occupation? Give your rationale. (Objective 4)

8. What factors are affecting the emergence of nursing as a profession? (Objective 4)

9. Do you believe nursing possesses a unique body of knowledge? Defend your answer. (Objective 4)

10. What is the importance of a code of ethics to a profession? What do you believe should be included in a code of ethics? (Objective 4)

11. Which of the criteria that an occupation must meet to be a profession do some persons believe nursing fails to meet? (Objective 4)

12. What educational preparation do you believe a nurse should possess in order to be considered a professional? Defend your answer. (Objectives 3 and 4)

13. In what way do you believe the increasing technology with which nurses must work affects the definition of nursing and the professionalization of the role? (Objectives 1 and 4)

14. Of the seven characteristics of a profession, which one do you believe is most lacking in nursing? Why? How important do you believe this to be? Why? (Objective 5)

15. What is meant by the term *body of specialized knowledge*? (Objective 5)

16. Do you think it is important for nursing education to take place in institutions of higher education? Why or why not? (Objective 5)

17. What do you see as the relationship between a code of ethics and professionalism? (Objective 5)

18. Discuss the concepts of altruism and service to the public in relationship to adequate salaries for nurses. (Objective 5)

19. Compare and contrast the terms *profession* and *professional*. (Objective 6)

20. In what ways are the sociological and legal definitions more restrictive than the popular definition of the term *professional*? (Objective 6)

21. Of the many media that influence nursing's image, which offer the most accurate portrayal? Why? (Objective 7)

22. Discuss the image of nursing today. Why are nurses concerned about it? (Objective 7)

23. Discuss the image of nursing as typically portrayed in novels. Has that image helped or hindered nursing? Why? (Objective 7)

24. Many of the early nursing studies focused on nursing curricula. Why do you think this happened? (Objective 8)

25. Of the many studies of nursing discussed in your textbook, select the one that you believe was the most important and tell why. (Objective 8)

26. The Pew Commission in 1995 recommended that scopes of practice be eliminated. How would that affect nursing? Do you believe it would have a positive or negative effect? Why?

27. Discuss the history of the nursing pin. (Objective 9)

28. Do you believe the nursing cap should be a standard part of the nursing uniform? Why or why not? (Objective 9)

29. Do you believe that nursing should continue to perpetuate such traditions as "pinning ceremonies"? Defend your answer. (Objective 9)

## FILL IN THE BLANKS

*Instructions: Complete the following statements by filling in the blanks with the word or words that make the sentence complete and correct.*

1. The definition of nursing and the role of the nurse have been significantly affected by _____ _____. (Objective 1)

2. The individual who defined the nurse's role as one that would "put the patient in the best condition for nature to act upon him" was _____ _____. (Objective 1)

3. The formulation of clear and concise definitions of nursing have been hampered by the lack of an obvious distinction between _____ and _____. (Objective 2)

4. In general, _____ is concerned with the diagnosis and treatment of disease. (Objective 2)

5. In general, _____ is concerned with caring for the person in a variety of health-related situations. (Objective 2)

6. The individual who was asked to write a definition of nursing for a committee of the International Council of Nurses was _____ _____. (Objective 3)

7. Two professional groups that have developed definitions of nursing are the _____ _____ _____ and the _____ _____ — _____ _____ __ _____. (Objective 3)

8. Another factor that has made it difficult to define nursing is that it is taught as encompassing both _____ and _____ aspects but is pursued primarily through practice. (Objective 1)

9. One of the early reports that focused on medicine but provided incentive for future efforts to define and discuss the characteristics of a profession was the _____ _____. (Objective 4)

10. A primary criticism leveled at nursing is that nursing has no _____ __ _____ _____. (Objectives 4 and 5)

11. One of the factors important in advancing the growth of the body of knowledge in nursing is the use of the _____ _____. (Objectives 4 and 5)

12. Two factors that result in an increase in nursing knowledge are _____ _____ and _____ _____. (Objectives 4 and 5)

13. Perhaps no issue in nursing has been more controversial than the _____ of its practitioners. (Objectives 4 and 5)

14. The ability of any group to function _____ has always been important to critics reviewing professions against professional standards. (Objective 4)

15. The general standard for the professional behavior of nurses in the United States is the _____ _____ ___ _____. (Objectives 4 and 5)

16. The _____ _____ __ _____ sets the standards for ethical practice by nurses throughout the world. (Objectives 4 and 5)

17. Some sociologists list as a characteristic of a profession that its members consider this to be their _____ _____. (Objective 4)

18. Today nurses recognize that "_____ _____" one's service should not be considered professional. (Objective 4)

19. Personal values result in a variation in the attributes that are considered _____. (Objective 6)

20. Federal legislation that has helped to establish a list of the characteristics of a professional is _____ _____ _____ - _____. (Objective 6)

21. To meet the nursing needs of the public, it is essential that caregivers function at various _____ _____ _____. (Objective 6)

22. The sociological and legal definitions are much more _____ than the popular definition of the term *professional*. (Objective 6)

23. Many nurses have been concerned that the _____ __ _____ does not accurately reflect the role of the professional nurse. (Objective 7)

24. In novels, nurses are almost always depicted as _____. (Objective 7)

25. The media that most accurately reflect the image of the nurse are _____ and _____. (Objective 7)

26. A consistently misrepresented image can negatively affect the way the _____ _____ ___ _____. (Objective 7)

27. The first nursing studies were not begun until the early _____. (Objective 8)

28. One of the earliest nursing studies was published by the U.S. Bureau of Education and was entitled ____
_____ _____ __ _____.
(Objective 8)

29. A study conducted in 1928 entitled "Nurses, Patients, and Pocket Books" was an inquiry into the _____ __ _____ __ _____. (Objective 8)

30. "Nursing for the Future," a study conducted by Esther Lucille Brown, recommended that nursing education be
_____ __ _____ __ _____ _____. (Objective 8)

31. A 5-year study conducted by Mildred Montag resulted in the establishment of
___ _____ _____ _____ _____.
(Objective 8)

32. A study, conducted in 1958 and entitled "Twenty-thousand Nurses Tell Their Story," looked at _____ __ _____ ____ _____ _____. (Objective 8)

33. The final report of the National Commission for the Study of Nursing and Nursing Education was entitled __ _____ __ _____. (Objective 8)

34. A 2-year study released in January 1983 was conducted by the Institute of Medicine Committee on Nursing and Nursing Education and was mandated by the ___ ____ ____ _____.
(Objective 8)

35. A group that sponsored many of the major studies of the 1990s was the _____ _____ _____. (Objective 8)

36. The tradition in nursing that may find its origin in the Crusades is the nursing _____. (Objective 9)

37. Many of the early nursing pins were fashioned after the _____ _____.
(Objective 9)

38. One of the early traditions of nursing that is seldom seen in nursing today is the _____. (Objective 9)

39. One of the traditions in nursing about which there is much discussion and some controversy is the _____.
(Objective 9)

40. One of the ceremonies that has become a tradition in nursing is the _____ that occurs at the completion of a program. (Objective 9)

## TRUE-FALSE QUESTIONS

*Instructions: Mark the following statements "T" if true or "F" if false. If using a scoring card, mark "A" if true or "B" if false.*

_____ 1. Most nurses have been able to agree on a single definition of nursing. (Objective 1)

_____ 2 Technological advances have affected the definition of nursing. (Objective 1)

_____ 3. The fact that the majority of nurses are women has had little effect on the definition of nursing. (Objective 1)

_____ 4. The fact that there are several educational routes to registered nursing has complicated the process of defining nursing. (Objective 1)

_____ 5. The scope of practice of nursing as defined in state practice acts is a critical factor in defining nursing. (Objective 1)

_____ 6. Nursing has always been concerned with the diagnosis and treatment of disease. (Objective 2)

_____ 7. The caring aspects of nursing are well documented in nursing literature. (Objective 2)

_____ 8. It makes little difference whether the public has clear information about nurses and nursing as long as they get good care. (Objective 2)

_____ 9. The terms *nurse* and *nursing* have been applied to a wide variety of health care activities, in many different settings, performed by people with a variety of educational backgrounds. (Objective 1)

_____ 10. Virginia Henderson provided a definition of nursing that is widely accepted throughout the world. (Objective 3)

_____ 11. Florence Nightingale emphasized the individual's need for self-care action in her definition of nursing. (Objective 3)

_____ 12. Martha Rogers advanced the concept of the unitary human in her definition of nursing. (Objective 3)

_____ 13. Sister Callista Roy's definition of nursing focused on interpersonal aspects. (Objective 3)

_____ 14. The American Nurses Association used the words *care, cure,* and *coordination* in identifying the essential components of professional practice. (Objective 3)

_____ 15. Nursing is primarily defined through the educational aspects of the profession. (Objectives 1 and 3)

_____ 16. "The Social Policy Statement" published by the ANA defines nursing as the diagnosis and treatment of human responses to health problems. (Objectives 1 and 3)

_____ 17. The single most important part of any nurse practice act is the legal definition of nursing practice. (Objectives 1 and 3)

_____ 18. Nursing leaders and theorists disagree as to whether nursing is a unique profession or one borrowed from other disciplines. (Objective 4)

_____ 19. It makes little difference to a profession, the manner in which its members approach growth and change. (Objective 4)

_____ 20. Most sociological definitions of a profession require that it possess a specialized body of knowledge. (Objective 4)

_____ 21. Most sociological definitions of a profession require that it provide the same education to all of its practitioners. (Objective 4)

_____ 22. Advances in nursing research and in nursing practice have had little effect on how the profession is viewed. (Objective 5)

_____ 23. Today, the majority of nursing programs preparing registered nurses are located in collegiate settings. (Objective 5)

_____ 24. The education of practitioners has been one of the few issues on which nurses have reached agreement. (Objective 5)

_____ 25. Controversy over the length of nursing education programs and the "technical" aspects of patient care continues. (Objective 5)

_____ 26. Most critics reviewing professions against professional standards place an emphasis on the ability of any group to function autonomously. (Objectives 4 and 5)

_____ 27. Today nursing and nurses have little input into policies and protocols and almost no accountability for practice. (Objective 5)

_____ 28. The general standard for professional behavior of nurses in the United States is the Nightingale Pledge. (Objective 6)

_____ 29. Nursing involves activities that may be performed by many different caregivers. (Objective 6)

_____ 30. The approach a person has to his or her role as a professional has little to do with the manner in which that discipline is viewed by others. (Objective 6)

_____ 31. Some people think that profession-alism has a great deal to do with attitude, dress, conduct, and deport-ment. (Objective 6)

_____ 32. In studying nurses on television, Kalisch and Kalisch found that nurses have substantive roles in television stories. (Objective 7)

_____ 33. Newspapers and news magazines tend to project the most accurate image of nursing today. (Objective 7)

_____ 34. The image of nursing was at its highest in the 1970s. (Objective 7)

_____ 35. One of the most recent studies conducted about nursing was done by Esther Lucille Brown and is enti-tled "Nursing for the Future." (Objective 8)

_____ 36. One of the issues frequently studied regarding nursing is the supply and demand for nurses. (Objective 8)

_____ 37. Early studies of nursing focused primarily on curriculum issues. (Objective 8)

_____ 38. Because nursing is a relatively young profession, it possesses few traditions. (Objective 9)

_____ 39. The actual symbolism of the nursing pin relates to customs established in the 16th century. (Objective 9)

_____ 40. The requirement for special dress in nursing came from the religious and military history of nursing. (Objective 9)

## MATCHING QUESTIONS

_Instructions: Match the numbered items with the most appropriate lettered items._

### Group A (Objective 1)

_____ 1. Developed a definition of nursing that emphasized unitary man.

_____ 2. Believed the goal of nursing was to place man in the best position for nature to act upon him.

_____ 3. Viewed nursing as an interpersonal process with a common goal of assisting the individual who is sick.

_____ 4. Employed a systems approach in her definition of nursing.

_____ 5. Focused a definition of nursing around 21 nursing problems.

_____ 6. Believed the goal of nursing was the promotion of adaptive responses.

   a. Florence Nighingale

   b. Faye Abdellah

   c. Dorothea Johnson

   d. Martha Rogers

   e. Sister Callista Roy

   f. Hildegard Peplau

### Group B (Objective 8)

_____ 1. Looked at what and how students were being taught.

_____ 2. Looked into the supply and demand for nurses.

_____ 3. Described the nursing schools of the period.

_____ 4. Studied the practices of over 1,000 nursing schools.

_____ 5. Looked at nurses, what they were doing, their attitudes and job satisfaction.

_____ 6. A report requested by the U.S. Surgeon General.

     a. "Twenty-thousand Nurses Tell Their Story"

     b. "The Educational Status of Nursing"

     c. "Toward Quality in Nursing: Needs and Goals"

     d. "Nurses, Patients, and Pocket Books"

     e. "Nursing Schools at the Mid-Century"

     f. "Winslow-Goldmark Report on Nursing and Nursing Education in the United States"

## Group C (Objective 4)

_____ 1. A characteristic of a profession that some say is lacking in nursing.

_____ 2. Should attract people of certain intellectual and personal qualities.

_____ 3. Entrusts the education of its practitioners to institutions of higher education.

_____ 4. Must have a strong internal organization of members.

_____ 5. A general standard for professional behavior.

_____ 6. Service to the public.

     a. Code of ethics

     b. Characteristic of a profession that has resulted in much controversy in nursing

     c. Similar to altruism

     d. Specialized body of knowledge

     e. Characteristic of a profession emphasized by Bixler and Bixler

     f. Characteristic of a profession identified by Flexner

## Group D (Objective 7)

_____ 1. The era when a great deal of time and energy was invested in studying the image of nursing.

_____ 2. The image of nursing in movies hit a high point during these years.

_____ 3. The image of nursing in movies hit a low point during these years.

_____ 4. "The English Patient" portrayed the nurse character as caring, thinking, and involved.

_____ 5. Books published during these years depicted a nurse with a hospital-based education.

_____ 6. Various nursing organizations waged campaigns to enhance the image of nursing.

     a. 1940s

     b. 1960s

     c. 1970s

     d. 1970s and 1980s

     e. 1980s

     f. 1997

## MULTIPLE-CHOICE QUESTIONS

_Instructions: Choose the one best answer for each question._

1. Which of the following is one reason why we have had difficulty defining nursing?

     a. The advancing technology in the health fields has changed the role of the nurse.

     b. Nurses have been unwilling to accept changing roles.

     c. The public is not responsive to defining nursing.

d. Hospital administrations block efforts to define nursing.

(Objective 1)

2. The "Social Policy Statement" that provided a definition of nursing was developed by which nursing organization?

   a. National League for Nursing

   b. American Nurses Association

   c. National Council of State Boards of Nursing

   d. National Student Nurse Association

   (Objective 1)

3. What is the single most important part of any Nurse Practice Act?

   a. Establishing a rate of pay for registered nurses

   b. Defining incompetent practice

   c. Establishing a legal definition of nursing practice

   d. Establishing the roles of the various members of the board

   (Objective 1)

4. Which of the following is one of the factors that has hampered the formulation of a clear and concise definition of nursing?

   a. Apathy on the part of nurses

   b. Fear of public response

   c. Interference by the medical profession

   d. Lack of an obvious distinction between nursing and medicine

   (Objective 2)

5. In general, nursing is concerned with which one of the following?

   a. The diagnosis and treatment of disease

   b. Caring for the person in a variety of health-related situations

   c. Assisting the person in making life choices

   d. Advising the person regarding health practices

   (Objective 2)

6. Which one of the following individuals defined the goal of nursing as putting the patient in the best condition for nature to act upon him?

   a. Faye Abdellah

   b. Myra Levine

   c. Florence Nightingale

   d. Ernestine Wiedenbach

   (Objective 3)

7. Which of the following defined nursing as concerned with the individual's need for self-care action?

   a. Virginia Henderson

   b. Florence Nightingale

   c. Ida Jean Orlando

   d. Dorothea Orem

   (Objective 3)

8. Which of the following defined nursing's role as assisting the individual to carry out those activities he would perform unaided if he had the necessary strength?

   a. Virginia Henderson

   b. Florence Nightingale

   c. Dorothea Orem

   d. Hildegard Peplau

   (Objective 3)

9. Which of the following defined nursing's goal as the promotion of adaptive responses?

   a. Dorothea Johnson

   b. Imogene King

   c. Myra Levine

d. Sister Callista Roy

(Objective 3)

10. Which of the following is credited with a definition of nursing involving the science of unitary man?

a. Florence Nightingale

b. Myra Levine

c. Mildred Montag

d. Martha Rogers

(Objective 3)

11. Which one of the following organizations identified care, cure, and coordination as major elements of nursing practice?

a. American Association of Nurse Anesthetists

b. American Nurses Association

c. National League for Nursing

d. National Council of State Boards of Nursing

(Objective 3)

12. Which of the following organizations is the author of the Model Nurse Practice Act?

a. American Nurses Association

b. National Council of State Boards of Nursing

c. National League for Nursing

d. North American Nursing Diagnosis Association

(Objective 3)

13. Which one of the following reports provided the incentive for future efforts to define and discuss the characteristics of a profession?

a. Flexner Report

b. Ginzberg Report

c. Study of the National Institute of Medicine

d. Winslow-Goldmark Report

(Objective 4)

14. Which one of the following would most authors include as a characteristic of a profession?

a. A profession licenses all its practitioners.

b. A profession should develop and enforce its own code of ethics.

c. A profession mandates continuing education for continued practice.

d. A profession limits the number of persons who can enter the profession.

(Objective 4)

15. Which one of the following is a characteristic of a profession that some believe nursing fails to meet?

a. All members are adequately reimbursed for their services.

b. Only the most creative and intelligent are allowed membership.

c. It punishes those who violate the code of ethics.

d. It possesses a body of specialized knowledge.

(Objective 4)

16. Which of the following is identified as an important characteristic of a profession?

a. It uses the scientific method to enlarge the body of knowledge.

b. It systematically evaluates itself against established criteria.

c. It requires continuing education of its members.

d. It legislates on behalf of its benefactors.

(Objective 4)

17. Which of the following is defined in a code of ethics?

    a. Issues related to withholding or withdrawing nutrition

    b. Issues related to collective bargaining

    c. The general standard for reimbursement of services

    d. The general standard for professional behavior

    (Objective 4)

18. With regard to professional policy, which of the following is becoming a common practice in today's society?

    a. Consumer representation on professional boards

    b. A decrease in professional licensing fees

    c. A decrease in the size of professional boards

    d. An interdisciplinary approach to professional boards

    (Objective 4)

19. Which of the following is most true regarding the professional activity of nurses?

    a. They may delegate any activities they wish.

    b. They have little role in the establishment of policies.

    c. They are accountable for the care given to their assigned patients.

    d. They may write some basic orders for patient care.

    (Objective 4)

20. Which one of the following is particularly true in nursing today?

    a. Most nurses leave the profession for more lucrative careers.

    b. The salaries nurses receive are dropping as the surplus of nurses increases.

    c. There is a greater likelihood that individuals will pursue additional educational degrees.

    d. Most nurses will leave the profession by the age of 47 because it is so stressful.

    (Objective 4)

21. Which of the following is most true of nursing today?

    a. Nursing involves activities that may be performed by any different caregivers.

    b. Nursing involves less technical skill than in earlier years.

    c. Nursing involves less critical thinking than in previous years.

    d. Nursing involves increased levels of education for all caregivers.

    (Objective 6)

22. When we consider the word *professional,* we find the popular definition to vary because of which of the following?

    a. The characteristics of a professional have never been clearly defined.

    b. The meaning of the term has changed dramatically over the years.

    c. The term has a very limited meaning.

    d. Different people view the attributes of a professional differently.

    (Objective 6)

23. During the late 1970s and the early 1980s, a great deal of time and energy was invested in which of the following?

    a. Developing associate degree programs

    b. Establishing mandatory licensure in all states

    c. Developing a uniform disciplinary code

    d. Studying the image of nursing

    (Objective 7)

24. How have most nurses been portrayed in novels?

    a. Married, female, and mothers

    b. Male, married, and under 35

    c. Single, female, and under 35

    d. Over 35, male or female, and married

    (Objective 7)

25. What have nurses done to discourage television advertisements or programs that portray nurses and nursing in a negative light?

    a. Boycott purchase of the items advertised

    b. Write to their legislator

    c. Ignore the reference to nursing

    d. Write to the consumer affairs department

    (Objective 7)

26. Why are nurses concerned about the image of nurses portrayed to the public?

    a. It will have an impact on the attitudes of prospective nurses.

    b. It will result in the public believing that nurses are overpaid.

    c. It will make it more difficult to find jobs in nursing.

    d. It creates dissension between nurses and physicians.

    (Objective 7)

27. In movies of the 1970s, few films centered on which of the following?

    a. Stories about nurses and nursing

    b. The individual achievement or personal autonomy of the nurse

    c. The role of the nurse in mental institutions

    d. Nurses' professional motivations and health care perspectives

    (Objective 7)

28. Which of the following images did Muff identify when she reviewed the image of nurses on get-well cards?

    a. Battle-axes

    b. Handmaiden

    c. Ministering angel

    d. Token torturer

    (Objective 7)

29. Who was the first nurse to be commemorated on a U.S. postage stamp because she volunteered to be bitten by the disease-carrying mosquito in an effort to determine how yellow fever was transmitted?

    a. Clara Barton

    b. Lavinia Dock

    c. Clara Maass

    d. Mary Mahoney

    (Objective 7)

30. In which of the following situations has the image of nursing typically been positive?

    a. During wartime

    b. During peacetime

    c. During nursing strikes

    d. During natural disasters

    (Objective 7)

31. Which of the following is a nursing organization that waged campaigns to enhance the image of nursing in the early 1980s?

    a. International Council of Nurses

    b. National Federation of Licensed Practical Nurses

c. National League for Nursing

d. National Student Nurse Association

(Objective 7)

32. What was the major focus of the earliest studies of nursing?

a. Nursing as a profession

b. Nursing education

c. Nursing practice

d. Nursing research

(Objective 8)

33. The study entitled "Twenty-thousand Nurses Tell Their Story" provided information regarding which one of the following?

a. Nursing salaries

b. Nursing curricula

c. Nurses themselves

d. Future nursing needs

(Objective 8)

34. Which of the following is a recommendation of the Institute of Medicine study?

a. More money be allocated to nursing education

b. The federal government discontinue efforts to increase the supply of "generalist nurses"

c. Nurses be required to have a baccalaureate degree to practice registered nursing

d. All nursing programs be run in conjunction with a medical school

(Objective 8)

35. Who conducted the study entitled "Nursing for the Future"?

a. Esther Lucille Brown

b. William Flexner

c. Jerome Lysaught

d. Mildred Montag

(Objective 8)

36. What was the title of one of the earliest (1912) studies of nursing?

a. "An Activity Analysis of Nursing"

b. "Nursing for the Future"

c. "Patterns of Patient Care"

d. "The Educational Status of Nursing"

(Objective 8)

37. Which study of nursing resulted in the establishment of associate degree nursing programs?

a. "Community College Education for Nursing"

b. "National Institute of Medicine Study"

c. "The Study of Credentialing in Nursing"

d. "Twenty-thousand Nurses Tell Their Story"

(Objective 8)

38. Who conducted a recent study entitled "Reforming Health Care Workforce Regulation"?

a. Kellogg Foundation

b. Department of Health Services

c. American Nurses Foundation

d. Pew Commission

(Objective 8)

39. Which of the following traditions in nursing found its origins in the Crusades?

a. Cap

b. Lamp

c. Pin

d. Uniform

(Objective 9)

40. Which of the following is true of the nursing pin?

    a. All graduates are required to purchase one.

    b. Each school has a unique pin.

    c. They will be eliminated after 2000.

    d. They were started to commemorate Civil War nurses.

    (Objective 9)

41. Which of the following is true with regard to the nurse's cap?

    a. It is a standard part of the nurse's uniform.

    b. It is required by public health policies.

    c. It has been dropped as a required article of dress in many hospitals.

    d. It should always be worn as a part of the uniform.

    (Objective 9)

# GAMING IN THE CLASSROOM

*Instructions: This game involves selecting teams and a host. The teams compete against one another for points. Each game has several subject categories. After teams are determined, a team is chosen to go first and selects a category. The host then poses the answer and the team provides the correct question for that answer. Each question can be awarded the same number of points or more difficult questions may be given heavier point values. (The instructor might determine which questions are more difficult based on the content emphasized in class.) Points are awarded to the team that is the first to signal and give a correct question. If that team is incorrect, the other team may attempt to provide the correct question and receive the points. The length of time allowed for response can be determined by the class or by the instructor. The team with the most points at the end of the game is declared the winner. Teams may be composed of individual students or groups of students. Teams may determine their answers as a team or may take turns answering as individuals.*

## Categories

A. Definitions of Nursing

B. Characteristics of a Profession

C. Image of Nursing

D. Studies about Nursing

E. Traditions in Nursing

## Answers and Questions

### Category A

A: Defined nursing's goal as putting the patient in the best condition for nature to act upon him.

Q: Who was Florence Nightingale?

A: Defined nursing's goal as the promotion of adaptive responses.

Q: Who was Sister Callista Roy?

A: Defined nursing around the science of unitary man.

Q: Who was Martha Rogers?

A: Defined nursing's role as assisting the individual to carry out those activities he would perform unaided if he had the necessary strength, will, or knowledge.

Q: Who was Virginia Henderson?

A: Defined nursing around 21 Nursing Problems.

Q: Who was Faye Abdellah?

### Category B

A: Nursing is frequently criticized as lacking this important characteristic.

Q: What is a body of specialized knowledge that belongs uniquely to nursing?

A: It is critical when professions grow and change.

Q: What is a systematic way of looking at data?

A: When one learns from experienced practitioners.

Q: What is an apprenticeship?

Q: A general standard for the professional behavior of nurses.

A: What is a code of ethics?

Q: The desire to provide for the good of society or service to the public.

A: What is altruism?

## Category C

A: The image of nursing reached an all time low during this time.

Q: What were the 1970s?

A: The media source that has most accurately reflected on nursing as a profession.

Q: What are newspapers and news magazines?

A: The nurse was almost always female, single, childless, white, and younger than 35.

Q: What was the image of nurses in novels?

A: A World War I heroine who was shot by the Germans for helping Allied soldiers escape.

Q: Who was Edith Cavell?

A: A malevolent and sadistic nurse from *One Flew Over the Cuckoo's Nest*.

Q: Who was Nurse Ratched?

## Category D

A: A 1970 study that looked at current practices and patterns of nursing.

Q: What was "An Abstract for Action"?

A: A study that resulted in the establishment of associate degree nursing programs.

Q: What was "Community College Education for Nursing"?

A: A study that was required by the Nursing Training Act of 1979.

Q: What was the "National Institute of Medicine Study"?

A: Looked at nurses, what they were doing, their attitudes toward their jobs, and job satisfaction.

Q: What was "Twenty-thousand Nurses Tell Their Story"?

A: A recent study that recommended reform of the licensing process.

Q: What was "Reforming Health Care Workforce Regulation"?

## Category E

A: Can find its origins in the Crusades.

Q: What is the nursing pin?

A: Many nurses have eliminated this as part of the nursing uniform.

Q: What is the cap?

A: A ceremony that has traditionally celebrated the completion of a nursing program.

Q: What is pinning?

A: Is an eight-pointed cross formed by four arrowheads joining at their points.

Q: What is the Maltese Cross?

A: Consisted of a bodice and skirt of white material, adjustable white cuffs, a stiff white collar, and a white cap.

Q: What is the typical uniform of early nursing schools?

A: Is often recited at pinning ceremonies.

Q: What is the Nightingale Pledge?

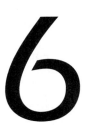

# Educational Preparation for Nursing

## PURPOSE

Chapter 6 discusses nursing education from a variety of perspectives. It outlines factors that have resulted in changes in nursing education, including the development of accreditation standards, the licensing examination, the changing role of the nurse, and some of the studies and reports that have focused on nursing. The activities that led up to the development of the American Nurses Association (ANA) position paper are discussed briefly, as well as the positions taken by other organizations. Problems encountered in implementing the position paper are outlined, with specific attention paid to the issues surrounding titling and the grandfather clause. The concept of differentiated practice is examined along with a discussion of competency statements. A discussion of the impact of federal funding for nursing education and a brief review of the major nursing theorists conclude the chapter.

## OBJECTIVES

1. Compare and contrast the educational preparation of the nursing assistant, the licensed practical (vocational) nurse, the graduate of a hospital-based program, the associate degree graduate, and the baccalaureate degree graduate.

2. Identify the purposes of other forms of nursing education: external degree programs, registered nurse baccalaureate programs, master's preparation, doctoral studies, and nondegree programs.

3. Discuss the concept of articulated programs.

4. Identify factors that have prompted change in nursing education, including studies and sociopolitical events.

5. Discuss the development and effect of the ANA position paper on nursing education, and the arguments for and against it.

6. Explain what is meant by a grandfather clause and the effect of such a clause on proposed changes in licensure.

7. Discuss the concept of differentiated practice and provide a rationale for its development.

8. Identify factors that have influenced changes in nursing education and explain the effect of each.

9. Analyze the ways in which nursing theories serve to advance the profession.

10. Define the continuing education unit, discuss its purpose, and identify the major points supporting mandatory continuing education and the major points supporting voluntary continuing education.

## KEY TERMS

Accreditation
Advanced placement
Advanced practice
Articulation
Associate degree
Baccalaureate degree education
Career ladder
Community based
Competencies
Differentiated practice
Diploma
Doctorate
Educational mobility
Entry into practice
External degree
Grandfather clause
Home health aide
Hospital-based program
Internship
Interstate endorsement
Mandatory continuing education
Nursing assistant
Position paper
Postsecondary education

Practical (vocational) nurse

Registered nurse

Scope of practice

Theorist/theory

Titling

Voluntary continuing education

## SITUATIONS TO FOSTER CRITICAL THINKING

1. If you were able to develop a plan for nursing education that would be adopted by the profession, what would that plan include? What testing mechanism would you put in place? How would you manage interstate endorsement? (Objectives 1 through 3)

2. Because nursing is producing so many variously educated nurses, how do you see each being used in nursing practice? Do you support so many levels of preparation? Why or why not? If you were to eliminate any level(s) which would it be? Give your rationale. (Objectives 2 and 7)

3. What do you see as the advantages of articulated programs? What are the disadvantages? What changes would you make in the process if you could? Why do you think those changes are important? (Objective 3)

4. Which factor do you believe has had the greatest impact on nursing education within the last 100 years. Give your rationale. (Objective 4)

5. Take a position with regard to the ANA position paper. Defend that position. (Objective 5)

6. Do you believe that grandfather clauses should be continued? Make a case for your answer. If you support grandfather clauses as they exist, give the reasons you believe some persons should unconditionally be allowed to continue to practice under old rules or regulations. If you believe grandfathering should be conditional, defend your position. How would you determine how long the conditional time should be? What would you recommend if the conditions were not met? (Objective 6)

7. Do you believe that hospitals should incorporate differentiated practice into their staffing patterns? Provide the rationale for your answer. Would you tie salary to the type of educational preparation for registered nurses? Why or why not? (Objective 7)

8. Do you believe that the federal government should continue to allocate money for nursing education? Why? If you believe it should, give reasons that you believe nursing should be given the funds when many other professions are not? If you believe it should not, what other mechanisms might be available to assist with the funding of nursing education? (Objective 8)

9. Select one of the nursing theories discussed in the text. Outline how it explains nursing as you believe it should be practiced. Why did you select that theory? Why do you think that theory is important to nursing? What weaknesses, if any, do you see in the theory? (Objective 9)

10. Take a position on mandatory or voluntary continuing education. Why do you believe it should be conducted as you believe? What would be the benefits? What would be the disadvantages? How would you monitor it? (Objective 10)

## DISCUSSION/ESSAY QUESTIONS

1. Describe the differences between associate degree nursing preparation for registered nursing and preparation at the baccalaureate level. (Objective 1)

2. Compare the educational preparation of the practical (vocational) nurse with that of the nurse prepared with an associate degree. What do you see as major differences? (Objective 1)

3. What were the factors that resulted in the development of programs to certify nursing assistants? (Objective 1)

4. Describe the factors that have resulted in the closure of many of the hospital-based programs. (Objective 1)

5. Identify some of the concerns with regard to registered nurse baccalaureate programs. How do you think some of those problems might be handled? (Objective 2)

6. Discuss the major benefits of articulated nursing programs. What would be the disadvantages? (Objective 3)

7. Discuss the factors that have been identified as major issues to be faced in multiple-entry, multiple-exit programs. (Objective 3)

8. Discuss one of the major recommendations of the Brown report and identify its significance to nursing as a profession. (Objective 4)

9. Discuss activities that occurred in the 1950s and resulted in changes in nursing. (Objective 4)

10. How did the development of uniform licensing affect nursing education? (Objective 4)

11. Do you believe that nursing schools should meet national standards (i.e., be accredited)? Why? (Objective 4)

12. What were the major assumptions on which the ANA position paper was based? (Objective 5)

13. What were the four positions outlined in the ANA position paper? (Objective 5)

14. Why do you believe the ANA position paper has not been implemented? (Objective 5)

15. In general, what has been the response of the various states and other nursing organizations to the ANA position paper? (Objective 5)

16. Discuss the position of the North Dakota Board of Nursing regarding educational requirements for licensure. (Objective 5)

17. Identify and discuss the major problems you see associated with changing the educational requirements for licensure. (Objectives 5 and 6)

18. What kinds of concerns surrounded the titling issue? (Objective 6)

19. What is meant by scope of practice and how is it affected by the entry-into-practice issue? (Objective 5)

20. Discuss the concept of the grandfather clause and the reasons it is necessary when some laws are changed. (Objective 6)

21. What is meant by interstate endorsement and under what circumstances can it occur? (Objective 6)

22. In what ways might changes in the educational requirements for licensure affect interstate endorsement processes? (Objective 6)

23. Discuss the problems associated with defining the competencies of graduates of the various programs. (Objective 7)

24. Discuss the concept of differentiated practice and explain how, if implemented, it might change nursing education in the future. (Objective 7)

25. If you were assigned the responsibility for differentiating practice, where would you begin? (Objective 7)

26. What special projects have been completed that seek to implement differentiated practice? How successful do you believe they have been? (Objective 7)

27. Discuss the forces for change in nursing education and identify the one that you believe will be most significant. Give the rationale for your selection. (Objective 8)

28. What changes might one anticipate in nursing education in the future and what would be the impetus for these changes? (Objective 8)

29. Describe how nursing benefited from federal funding in the past. (Objective 8)

30. In what ways do you believe increasing emphasis on educational mobility will affect nursing education? (Objective 8)

31. What are the factors that have led to the increase in community-based nursing? How do you see that changing the education for nurses? (Objective 8)

32. In what ways do you see the computer used in nursing? Do you believe you are receiving adequate preparation for this in your program? (Objective 8)

33. What is meant by a theory of nursing? (Objective 9)

34. Why has the development of nursing theories flourished in the nursing profession? (Objective 9)

35. Identify some of the nursing theorists who have developed nursing theories that speak to the art and science of humanistic nursing. (Objective 9)

36. Identify some nursing theorists who have developed nursing theories that involve interpersonal relationships. (Objective 9)

37. Identify some nursing theorists who have developed systems theories. (Objective 9)

38. What role do you see nursing theories playing in the development of nursing as a profession? (Objective 9)

39. Do you believe continuing education in nursing should be mandatory? Defend your position. (Objective 10)

40. What are some of the problems associated with mandating continuing education for licensure? (Objective 10)

# FILL IN THE BLANKS

*Instructions: Complete the following statements by filling in the blanks with the word or words that make the sentence complete and correct.*

1. In 1987, Congress passed the _____ _____ ___, which includes the regulation of education and certification of nursing assistants who work in nursing homes. (Objective 1)

2. A popular belief regarding practical (vocational) nursing programs is that they were initiated through the _____ in Brooklyn, New York, around 1892. (Objective 1)

3. Practical nursing programs expanded rapidly during the _____. (Objective 1)

4. The earliest type of nursing education in the United States took place in _____ programs administered by hospitals. (Objective 1)

5. The movement toward associate degree education began in _____. (Objective 1)

6. The advent of associate degree education in nursing has brought with it greater _____ in the students who enroll in nursing programs. (Objective 1)

7. One of the major challenges to associate degree nursing programs is the inclusion of _____ _____ _____. (Objective 1)

8. The first school of nursing to be established in a university setting was started at the University of Minnesota in ____. (Objective 1)

9. One of the components offered in baccalaureate programs that is not present in most other programs is an introduction to _____. (Objective 1)

10. The concept of the generic master's program was developed at _____. (Objective 1)

11. One of the similarities of all programs preparing registered nurses is that the graduates all take the same _____ _____. (Objective 1)

12. The programs established to provide a baccalaureate degree to nurses who are already licensed as registered nurses are called _____ _____ _____ programs. (Objective 2)

13. The concept of the external degree is based on assessment of learning through _____and _____ examinations. (Objective 2)

14. The purpose of articulated programs is for students to start at one level and continue _____ ____ _____. (Objective 3)

15. A report on nursing prepared by Esther Lucile Brown was titled _____ ____ ____ _____. (Objective 4)

16. The professional nursing group that is responsible for accrediting nursing programs is the _____. (Objective 4)

17. The first position taken by the ANA position paper states that the education for all who practice nursing should take place in _____ ___ _____. (Objective 5)

18. According to the ANA position paper, the minimum educational preparation to practice professional nursing should be a (an) _____ _____. (Objective 5)

19. According to the ANA position paper, the minimum educational preparation to practice technical nursing should be a (an) _____ _____. (Objective 5)

20. As of January 1987, a baccalaureate degree is required for registered nursing in the state of _____. (Objective 5)

21. The section of the Nurse Practice Act that outlines the activities a person with that license may perform is referred to as the _____ ___ _____. (Objective 5)

22. When a state licensure law is changed, a _____ clause has been a standard feature that allows persons to continue to practice their occupation after new qualifications have been enacted into law. (Objective 6)

23. Two of the major issues surrounding the ANA position paper involve _____ and _____. (Objective 5)

24. The process that allows a nurse who has written and passed the licensure examination in one state to move to another and obtain a license without retaking the examination is known as _____ _____. (Objective 5)

25. Moving toward differentiated practice would require defining the _____ of graduates of the various types of nursing education programs. (Objective 7)

26. Graduates of baccalaureate nursing programs, associate degree programs, and hospital-based programs all write the same _____ _____. (Objective 7)

27. One of the challenges to nursing educators has been the growing emphasis on _____ _____ in nursing. (Objective 8)

28. A significant change in nursing practice is the trend toward _____ practice. (Objective 8)

29. A major technological advance that we see in health care and also in nursing education programs is the increasing use of _____. (Objective 8)

30. The bases for hypotheses about nursing practice may be found in nursing _____. (Objective 9)

31. The nursing theory developed by Sister Callista Roy is known as a (an) _____ theory. (Objective 9)

32. The nursing theory developed by Betty Neuman might be identified as _____ theory. (Objective 11)

33. The nursing theory known as the science of unitary man was developed by _____ _____. (Objective 9)

34. Dorothy Orem's theory of nursing focuses on the concept of _____. (Objective 9)

35. The individual noted for her development of a definition of nursing is _____ _____. (Objective 9)

36. Theories that deal with interactions between and among individuals are known as _____ theories. (Objective 9)

37. A planned learning experience beyond a basic nursing educational program is known as _____ _____. (Objective 10)

38. It has been suggested that the first continuing education programs in nursing were initiated at _____ _____ at _____ _____. (Objective 10)

39. A rather uniform system of measuring, recording, reporting, and recognizing continuing education in nursing is through _____ _____ _____. (Objective 10)

40. The main goal of continuing education for nurses is to ensure that they remain _____ __ _____. (Objective 10)

## TRUE-FALSE QUESTIONS

*Instructions: Mark the following statements "T" if true or "F" if false. If using a scoring card, mark "A" if true or "B" if false.*

_____ 1. In 1987, Congress passed the Omnibus Budget Reconciliation Act, which regulates agencies receiving federal funds including regulations regarding the education and certification of nursing assistants. (Objective 1)

_____ 2. The skills that may be performed by the nursing assistant are determined by the National Council of State Boards of Nursing. (Objective 1)

_____ 3. Practical nurse education is the newest form of nursing education in the United States and Canada. (Objective 1)

_____ 4. Practical nurse education programs rapidly expanded as a result of World War II. (Objective 1)

_____ 5. The general curriculum of the practical nurse programs takes approximately 18 months for completion. (Objective 1)

_____ 6. The practical nurse programs, as designed today, are incompatible with the career ladder concept. (Objective 1)

_____ 7. The earliest type of nursing education in the United States took place in diploma programs administered by hospitals. (Objective 1)

_____ 8. The length of hospital-based programs varies in length today from 36 to 48 months. (Objective 1)

_____ 9. Since the 1960s there has been a significant decline in the number of hospital-based programs. (Objective 1)

_____ 10. Associate degree nursing programs have the distinction of being the first type of nursing education established on the basis of planned research and experimentation. (Objective 1)

_____ 11. Most associate degree programs are located in 4-year colleges and universities. (Objective 1)

_____ 12. The recent shift to community-based practice offers a challenge to associate degree educators. (Objective 1)

_____ 13. The concept of the associate degree in nursing is well understood by employers and the public. (Objective 1)

_____ 14. The first school of nursing to be established in a university setting was started at the University of Minnesota in 1909. (Objective 1)

_____ 15. Most of the early programs offering a baccalaureate degree were limited to 4 years in length. (Objective 1)

_____ 16. Many nursing leaders have advocated for baccalaureate education as the minimum educational preparation for supervisory and administrative nursing roles. (Objective 1)

_____ 17. The accreditation standards governing baccalaureate nursing programs require that all programs include a component dealing with specialization. (Objective 1)

_____ 18. The concept of a master's degree in nursing that would lead to nursing licensure was developed at Yale University and several other universities. (Objective 1)

_____ 19. One of the reasons educational offerings in nursing have expanded tremendously since the 1960s is the result of the changing role of the nurse in health care delivery. (Objective 2)

_____ 20. Registered nurse baccalaureate programs throughout the United States are very much the same. (Objective 2)

_____ 21. A concern in registered nurse baccalaureate programs is determining what credit should be granted for previous education. (Objective 2)

_____ 22. The critical need for nurses with additional preparation to work in educational settings and in supervisory roles has resulted in more programs at the graduate level. (Objective 2)

_____ 23. The number of requests for admission to doctoral study in nursing has greatly decreased since the early 1980s. (Objective 2)

_____ 24. The purpose of an articulated program is to facilitate opportunities for students to start nursing education, stop when some goal is achieved, or keep moving up the educational ladder. (Objective 3)

_____ 25. No programs exist that provide articulation between practical nurse programs and registered nurse programs because of differences in scopes of practice. (Objective 3)

_____ 26. Recent health care reform has resulted in an increased emphasis on the role of advanced nursing practice in health care delivery. (Objective 3)

_____ 27. The Brown report emerged because of concern for the fact that young women were not choosing nursing as a profession. (Objective 4)

_____ 28. Changes in nursing practice have required nurses prepared with higher levels of education. (Objective 4)

_____ 29. The report of the Surgeon General's Consultant Group found that the supply of nurses was adequate. (Objective 5)

_____ 30. The Nurse Training Act of 1964 was an outgrowth of the Surgeon General's report. (Objective 5)

_____ 31. As early as the 1950s, the ANA was concerned about the education for professional nursing. (Objective 5)

_____ 32. The ANA position paper on nursing education was first published in 1982. (Objective 5)

_____ 33. The ANA position paper on nursing education advocates a master's degree in nursing for the practice of professional nursing. (Objective 5)

_____ 34. The ANA position paper on nursing education proposes that all educational preparation for nursing occur in institutions of higher education. (Objective 5)

_____ 35. The ANA position paper on nursing education advocates that the minimum educational preparation for technical nursing be an associate degree in nursing. (Objective 5)

_____ 36. The ANA position paper on nursing education is based on an assumption that the demand for services of nurses will decrease. (Objective 5)

_____ 37. Most nursing organizations are not supportive of the concept of requiring a baccalaureate degree for professional nursing practice. (Objective 5)

_____ 38. The National Council of State Boards of Nursing has taken a formal position of neutrality on changes in nursing education requirements for entry. (Objective 5)

_____ 39. The state of North Dakota now requires a baccalaureate degree in nursing to allow graduates to write the licensure examination for registered nursing. (Objectives 5 and 6)

_____ 40. The National Federation of Licensed Practical Nurses has supported the concept of increasing the 1-year program to 18 months. (Objective 5)

_____ 41. The National Federation of Licensed Practical Nurses supports the use of the title "associate nurse" for the graduate of the practical nurse programs of the future. (Objective 5)

_____ 42. The titles to be used by persons working at each level have been identified by most states. (Objective 5)

_____ 43. The scope of practice is that section of the Nurse Practice Act that outlines the activities a person with that license may engage in legally. (Objective 5)

_____ 44. When a state licensure law is changed, the grandfather clause allows persons to continue to practice their profession after new qualifications they might not have met have been enacted into law. (Objective 6)

_____ 45. The scope of practice for the professional and that for the technical nurse are clearly defined and differentiated. (Objective 7)

_____ 46. Realistic statements regarding competencies of each level or category of nursing education are necessary so that each category of graduate can be used effectively and efficiently. (Objective 7)

_____ 47. There have been no projects initiated, to date, to attempt to differentiate statements of scope of practice. (Objective 7)

_____ 48. One of the recommendations of the recent Pew Commission was the strengthening of existing career ladder programs. (Objective 8)

_____ 49. Computer literacy among students and faculty is no longer an issue. (Objective 8)

_____ 50. Most nursing theories have little applicability to the actual practice of nursing. (Objective 9)

_____ 51. Nursing theories are usually classified with regard to the structure or approach around which they are developed. (Objective 9)

_____ 52. Stress adaptation models are based on concepts that view interactions between and among all the factors in a situation. (Objective 9)

_____ 53. One of the most recent classification of theories focuses on growth and development of the individual. (Objective 9)

_____ 54. Evidence of continuing education is a requirement for licensure renewal in all states except one. (Objective 10)

_____ 55. A system for accreditation and approval of continuing education in nursing was developed and implemented by the ANA in 1975.

## MATCHING QUESTIONS

*Instructions: Match the numbered items with the most appropriate lettered items.*

### Group A (Objectives 4, 5, and 8)

_____ 1. National League for Nursing

_____ 2. State Board of Nursing

_____ 3. National Federation of Licensed Practical Nurses

_____ 4. American Nurses Association

_____ 5. Surgeon General's Consultant Group on Nursing

_____ 6. State Board Test Pool Examination

    a. Developed a position paper on nursing education

    b. Has the responsibility for accrediting nursing programs

    c. Made recommendations regarding loans and scholarships for nursing students

    d. Helped all schools to focus on common goals and laid the foundation of interstate endorsement

    e. Is the organization that licenses nurses

    f. Supported the concept of an associate degree for licensed practical nurses

### Group B (Objective 9)

_____ 1. Unitary man

_____ 2. Adaptation

_____ 3. Self-care concept

_____ 4. Looked at total response of the person to the interaction between the internal and external environment

_____ 5. Health care systems model

_____ 6. Transcultural approach

    a. Madeleine Leininger

    b. Sister Callista Roy

    c. Myra Levine

    d. Martha Rogers

    e. Betty Newman

    f. Dorothy Orem

### Group C (Objectives 4, 5, and 8)

_____ 1. "Definition of Nursing"

_____ 2. "A Position Paper on Educational Preparation for Nurse Practitioners and Associates to Nurses"

_____ 3. "Defining and Differentiating ADN and BSN Competencies"

_____ 4. "Core, Care, and Cure Model"

_____ 5. "Twenty-one Nursing Problems"

_____ 6. "Transcultural Care Theory"

    a. American Nurses Association

    b. Lydia Hall

    c. Faye Abdellah

    d. Madeleine Leininger

    e. Midwest Alliance in Nursing (MAIN)

    f. Virginia Henderson

### Group D (Objective 1)

_____ 1. Occurs in 4-year schools and universities

_____ 2. Mandated through OBRA

_____ 3. Based on research and experimentation

_____ 4. The oldest form of nursing education in the United States

_____ 6. Implements the "ladder" concept

    a. Associate degree nursing education

    b. Articulated programs

c. Baccalaureate degree nursing education

d. Diploma programs

e. Nursing assistants

f. Registered nurse baccalaureate programs

# MULTIPLE-CHOICE QUESTIONS

*Instructions: Choose the one best answer for each question.*

1.  What are the minimum number of hours of theory required in the preparation of a nursing assistant?

    a. 25

    b. 50

    c. 75

    d. 100

    (Objective 1)

2.  Where did the first programs to offer formal preparation for practical nursing begin?

    a. Junior colleges

    b. State universities

    c. YWCA

    d. Churches

    (Objective 1)

3.  Who established the first accrediting service for practical nursing programs?

    a. American Nurses Association

    b. National League for Nursing

    c. National Federation of Licensed Practical Nurses

    d. Association of Practical Nurses Education and Service

    (Objective 1)

4.  In which states is the practical nurse known by the title *vocational* nurse?

    a. California and Texas

    b. Montana and Utah

    c. North Carolina and South Carolina

    d. New York and New Jersey

    (Objective 1)

5.  What is the period of study for most practical nurse programs?

    a. 6 months

    b. 9 months to 1 year

    c. 18 months

    d. 24 months

    (Objective 1)

6.  What type of nursing program might be located in a high school, trade or technical school, hospital, junior or community college, or independent agency?

    a. Nursing assistant or practical nurse program

    b. Associate degree program

    c. Baccaluareate degree program

    d. Master's degree program

    (Objective 1)

7.  Where were the earliest schools of nursing located?

    a. Community colleges

    b. Hospitals

    c. Senior colleges and universities

    d. Vocational-technical institutes

    (Objective 1)

8.  Where are diploma programs located?

    a. Community colleges

    b. Hospitals

    c. Technical-vocational institutes

d. Universities

(Objective 1)

9. How long is the traditional diploma program?

a. 1 year

b. 2 years

c. 3 years

d. 4 years

(Objective 1)

10. Where are associate degree nursing programs usually located?

a. Community colleges

b. Hospitals

c. Vocational-technical institutes

d. Universities

(Objective 1)

11. Who was the architect for associate degree nursing education?

a. Esther Lucille Brown

b. Virginia Henderson

c. Madeleine Leininger

d. Mildred Montag

(Objective 1)

12. Which type of nursing program describes its graduates as "skilled in bedside nursing"?

a. Associate degree

b. Baccalaureate

c. Nursing assistant

d. Vocational nursing

(Objective 1)

13. Where are baccalaureate nursing programs located?

a. Community colleges

b. Hospitals

c. Universities

d. Vocational-technical institutes

(Objective 1)

14. Which type of nursing program provides a basis for jobs in school nursing?

a. Associate degree programs

b. Baccalaureate degree programs

c. Hospital-based programs

d. Vocational-technical programs

(Objective 1)

15. In what year was the first baccalaureate nursing program started at the University of Minnesota?

a. 1853

b. 1875

c. 1909

d. 1922

(Objective 1)

16. At which level of nursing education does specialization occur?

a. Associate degree

b. Baccalaureate degree

c. Diploma

d. Master's degree

(Objective 2)

17. What is the name used to refer to programs that provide baccalaureate education to registered nurses?

a. Basic programs

b. External degree programs

c. Ladder programs

d. RNB programs

(Objective 2)

18. To what does the term *RNB* refer to?

a. 2-year generic programs

b. 4-year generic programs

c. Programs that provide baccalaureate education to registered nurses

d. Programs that require a step-by-step progression

(Objective 2)

19. Which of the following is one of the major problems associated with RNB programs?

    a. The accreditation of the program

    b. The large number of applicants

    c. The evaluation of previous learning

    d. The qualifications of the faculty

    (Objective 2)

20. The critical need for nurses to fulfill the expanded role of the nurse has resulted in the increase of which type of program?

    a. Associate degree

    b. Baccalaureate degree

    c. Master's degree

    d. Doctoral degree

    (Objective 2)

21. Which of the following statements is true of doctoral programs in nursing?

    a. Doctorates can be earned only in allied areas such as anthropology or education.

    b. Doctorates in nursing are increasing.

    c. Doctorates in nursing are decreasing.

    d. Doctorates in nursing are required for all leadership positions.

    (Objective 2)

22. Which type of program has no prescribed methods of learning and assesses learning through highly standardized and validated examinations?

    a. An articulated program

b. An external degree program

c. An open curriculum

d. Self-paced learning

(Objective 2)

23. What is the term used to refer to programs that allow an individual to move smoothly from one level of nursing education to the next with minimal loss of earned credit?

    a. Articulated programs

    b. External degree programs

    c. RNB programs

    d. Self-paced programs

    (Objective 3)

24. Articulated programs may also be known as which of the following?

    a. Continuing education programs

    b. External degree programs

    c. Internships

    d. Two-on-two programs

    (Objective 3)

25. Which program prepares the graduate for licensure?

    a. Articulated program

    b. Generic program

    c. Graduate program

    d. Two-on-two program

    (Objective 2)

26. Which of the following studies was published in the 1950s and had a significant impact on nursing?

    a. Brown report

    b. Flexner report

    c. Goldberg report

    d. Surgeon General's report

    (Objective 4)

27. Which of the following was a recommendation of the Brown report?

    a. That nursing move away from the system of apprenticeship that predominated at the time

    b. That nursing education be federally funded

    c. That a master's degree be required of all faculty

    d. That admissions to the nursing classes be limited

    (Objective 4)

28. When was the Brown study conducted?

    a. Right after World War I

    b. Right after World War II

    c. After the Korean conflict

    d. After the Vietnam conflict

    (Objective 4)

29. What was a recommendation of the Surgeon General's report?

    a. More financial assistance be provided for nursing education

    b. Roles of variously prepared graduates be differentiated

    c. More studies be conducted on the nursing shortage

    d. Associate degree nursing programs be closed

    (Objective 4)

30. Which of the following has created much discussion and dissension in nursing?

    a. Publication of the ANA Position on Nursing Education

    b. Publication of the Brown report

    c. Establishment of nursing assistant programs

    d. Publication of the Surgeon General's Report

    (Objective 5)

31. When was the ANA position paper published?

    a. 1942

    b. 1950

    c. 1965

    d. 1972

    (Objective 5)

32. Which of the following was based on the belief that improvement of nursing practice depended on the advancement of nursing education?

    a. ANA position paper

    b. Surgeon General's report

    c. Brown report

    d. Goldmark report

    (Objective 5)

33. Which of the following developed the ANA position paper?

    a. Committee on Education

    b. Committee on Economic Welfare

    c. Committee on Accreditation

    d. Committee on Standards of Education

    (Objective 5)

34. Which of the following statements accurately reflects one of the four positions taken in the ANA position paper?

    a. All of the current forms of nursing education should be continued.

    b. All education for nursing should occur in 4-year schools.

    c. The education for all who practice nursing should take place in institutions of higher education.

    d. The education of assistants in health care should be discontinued.

    (Objective 5)

35. The ANA position paper advocated which one of the following degrees or certificates as mandatory for entry into professional practice?

    a. Master's degree

    b. Bachelor's degree

    c. Associate degree

    d. Diploma

    (Objective 5)

36. The ANA position paper presented which of the following concerns?

    a. Mobility for nurses

    b. Job placement

    c. Articulated nursing programs

    d. Recruitment of faculty

    (Objective 5)

37. Which state now requires a baccalaureate degree in nursing in order to write the registered nursing licensing examinations?

    a. California

    b. Washington

    c. North Dakota

    d. New Hampshire

    (Objective 5)

38. What is one of the major problems associated with the ANA position paper?

    a. Salary of nurses

    b. Rights of nurses to bargain collectively

    c. Continuing education of nurses

    d. Titling of graduates of the different programs

    (Objective 5)

39. Which of the following statements is true of the grandfather clause?

    a. The grandfather clause has been a standard feature that allows persons to continue to practice their profession after new qualifications are enacted into law.

    b. The grandfather clause was mandated in legislation passed when the Supreme Court reached a decision on the Galt case.

    c. The grandfather clause is applicable to blue-collar occupations but not to nursing.

    d. The grandfather clause will expire by the year 1994, so nursing should make any needed changes soon.

    (Objective 6)

40. Which of the following features allows persons to continue to practice their profession after new qualifications that they might not meet have been enacted into law?

    a. Waiver

    b. Grandfather clause

    c. Immunity clause

    d. Granted release

    (Objective 6)

41. What is the process by which nurses licensed in one state can gain licensure in another state without reexamination?

    a. Transferability

    b. Protractability

    c. Extendibility

    d. Interstate endorsement

    (Objective 6)

42. Which of the following was the thrust of the Healing Web Project?

    a. Continuing education

    b. Differentiated practice

    c. Graduate education

    d. Recertification

    (Objective 7)

43. Which of the following represents a group that has worked at differentiating practice?

    a. ANA

    b. Council of State Boards

    c. Midwest Alliance in Nursing

    d. Surgeon General's Group

    (Objective 7)

44. Which of the following skills is most likely to be expected of all nurses of tomorrow?

    a. Ability to perform venipuncture

    b. Ability to read electroencephalogram strips

    c. Ability to interpret fetal monitor tracings

    d. Ability to operate a computer

    (Objective 8)

45. What is one of the major challenges facing nursing today?

    a. Setting accreditation standards

    b. Attracting men into the profession

    c. Describing and differentiating the competencies of graduates of various programs

    d. Establishing faculty workloads

    (Objective 7)

46. Nursing in the future may well require that all nurses possess which of the following?

    a. The ability to speak at least two languages

    b. Understanding of accounting principles

    c. Computer literacy

    d. Calculus skills

    (Objective 8)

47. One of the changes we are beginning to see in nursing education is the advent of programs that have been designed to do which of the following?

    a. Meet the needs of the adult learner

    b. Provide for greater structure in the program of learning

    c. Make more electives available to students

    d. Move students more rapidly through the program

    (Objective 8)

48. Which of the following is a significant change in nursing practice?

    a. Community-based practice

    b. The use of all-registered nurse staffing

    c. The revival of the functional nursing approach

    d. Longer hospital stays

    (Objective 8)

49. Nursing educators are revising programs of study to address the needs of which of the following?

    a. Economically disadvantaged students

    b. Hospital administration

    c. The new high school graduate

    d. The adult learner

    (Objective 8)

50. Which one of the following individuals developed a theory of nursing built around the concept of adaptation?

    a. Martha Rogers

    b. Betty Neuman

    c. Dorothy Orem

    d. Sister Callista Roy

    (Objective 9)

51. Which of the following individuals developed a theory of nursing around the concept of self-care?

    a. Martha Rogers

    b. Betty Neuman

    c. Dorothy Orem

    d. Sister Callista Roy

    (Objective 9)

52. Which of the following individuals is credited with advocating a transcultural approach to nursing theory?

    a. Martha Rogers

    b. Betty Neuman

    c. Madeleine Leininger

    d. Myra Levine

    (Objective 9)

53. What is the term used for planned learning experiences beyond a basic nursing educational program?

    a. Continuing education in nursing

    b. Post-baccalaureate nursing education

    c. Generic master's programs

    d. Preceptorships

    (Objective 10)

54. One of the issues in nursing today focuses around whether continuing education should:

    a. Be given college credit

    b. Be mandatory

    c. Require a clinical component

    d. Be totally eliminated

    (Objective 10)

55. Which organization is responsible for accrediting continuing education programs in nursing?

    a. ANA

    b. Council of State Boards

    c. NLN

    d. Department of Health Services

    (Objective 10)

# GAMING IN THE CLASSROOM

*Instructions: This game involves selecting teams and a host. The teams compete against one another for points. Each game has several subject categories. After teams are determined, a team is chosen to go first and selects a category. The host then poses the answer and the team provides the correct question for that answer. Each question can be awarded the same number of points or more difficult questions may be given heavier point values. (The instructor might determine which questions are more difficult based on the content emphasized in class.) Points are awarded to the team that is the first to signal and give a correct question. If that team is incorrect, the other team may attempt to provide the correct question and receive the points. The length of time allowed for response can be determined by the class or by the instructor. The team with the most points at the end of the game is declared the winner. Teams may be composed of individual students or groups of students. Teams may determine their answers as a team or may take turns answering as individuals.*

## Categories

A. Routes to Nursing Education

B. Similarities in Programs Preparing Graduates for Licensure

C. Entry-into-Practice Issues

D. Factors Affecting Nursing Education

E. Forces for Change in Nursing

## Answers and Questions

### Category A

A: Occurs predominately in community colleges.

Q: What is associate degree education?

A: The programs typically include public health experience.

Q: What is baccalaureate degree education?

A: Was the earliest type of nursing education in the United States.

Q: What is hospital-based (diploma) education?

A: The early programs started in the YWCA.

Q: What were practical (vocational) nursing programs?

A: Responds to the need for advanced practitioners in nursing.

Q: What are master's degrees in nursing?

### Category B

A: The requirement all graduates must meet if they wish to be registered nurses.

Q: What is passing the National Council Licensing Examination for registered nursing?

A: A factor that has made recruitment of nursing faculty an ongoing problem.

Q: What are lower salaries in education that lag behind those in practice?

A: A characteristic found among nursing students today.

Q: What is greater diversity (or similar words)?

A: A factor facing most admission departments in nursing programs.

Q: What is more applicants than seats available in a sound educational program?

A: A factor affecting the financial situation for students.

Q: What are increasing tuition costs?

### Category C

A: The titling of graduates from each of the different educational programs.

Q: What is one of the most controversial problems associated with changing requirements for licensure?

A: Outlines the activities a person with a particular license may legally perform.

Q: What is the scope of practice?

A: Allows persons to continue to practice their profession after new qualifications have been enacted into law.

Q: What is a grandfather clause?

A: Allows individuals licensed in one state to move to another state and practice there.

Q: What is interstate endorsement?

A: Registered associate nurse.

Q: What is one title suggested for the associate degree graduate?

### Category D

A: The report of a study of nursing conducted in 1948.

Q: What was the Brown report?

A: A report that emphasized the need for more nurses and identified the lack of adequate financial resources for nursing education as a major problem.

Q: What was the Report of the Surgeon General's Consultant Group?

A: Recommended that the minimum education for beginning profession nursing practice be baccalaureate education in nursing.

Q: What is a recommendation of the ANA position on nursing education?

A: Changed in response to changes in the workplace.

Q: What is the nurses' role (or similar words)?

A: Has created controversy and dissension in nursing for over 40 years.

Q: What is the response to the ANA position paper on nursing education?

## Category E

A: A trend toward community-based practice.

Q: What is a change in nursing practice occurring within the last few years?

A: A skill all graduates of the future will be expected to possess.

Q: What is the ability to use a computer?

A: The term referring to the ability to move from one level of education to another with minimal repetition of work.

Q: What is educational mobility?

A: The strengthening of existing career ladder programs.

Q: What is one of the recommendations of the Pew Commission?

A: Has resulted in more patients being cared for in their homes.

Q: What is early hospital discharge?

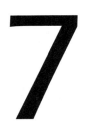

# Credentials for Health Care Providers

## PURPOSE

This chapter acquaints students with the various credentials used by individuals in the health care field. The discussion includes credentials in nursing, the history of their development, and the role that credentials play in the profession. It explores nursing licensure, what it means, who controls it, and how it affects the individual who wishes to practice nursing. Information regarding the disciplinary process for licensed professionals is presented. Issues surrounding the use of additional credentials such as certification are also discussed.

## OBJECTIVES

1. Define and discuss the concept of credentialing.

2. Differentiate among a diploma, certification, accreditation, and licensure as credentials.

3. Outline the history of nursing licensure including the concepts of permissive and mandatory licensure.

4. Identify the major topics found in nursing practice acts.

5. Outline the role of the State Board of Nursing or other state regulatory authority.

6. Differentiate between licensure by examination and licensure by endorsement.

7. Discuss the disciplinary process in regard to a nursing license.

8. Discuss the process of nursing licensure for graduates of foreign nursing schools.

9. Explain the various uses for certification in nursing.

10. Discuss current trends in credentialing within the health care workforce.

## KEY TERMS

Accreditation
Computerized adaptive testing
Credentialing
Disciplinary action
Grandfathering
License
Licensure by endorsement

Mandatory licensure
NCLEX-PN
NCLEX-RN
Permissive licensure
Scope of practice
Sunset laws

## SITUATIONS TO FOSTER CRITICAL THINKING

1. Several nurses on your unit would like to see a change made in the Nursing Practice Act in your state. You have been asked to gather information regarding the steps that should be taken to initiate a change. Where would you begin? Who would you write or telephone? Give the rationale for why you included the persons or organizations you have identified. How long might you expect the process to take? (Objective 5 and Chapter 3 objectives)

2. Do you believe the Nursing Practice Act for your state should include provisions for expanded practice? Provide a rationale for your answer. If you believe it should not, what group do you believe should oversee expanded practice? Why? Provide a rationale for your answer. (Objectives 4, 9, and 10)

3. Grace Barker is completing the registered nurse program at Rio Santiago College in California. She plans to get married and move with her husband to Illinois. She plans to work in Illinois while he completes his education. What options are available to Grace with regard to securing a license in Illinois? Which option would you advise her to pursue? What is the rationale for your answer? Where should she write or call for information? (Objectives 5 and 6)

4. Now that licensing examinations are computerized, do you think computerized simulation testing (CST) will be adopted in the future? What would you see as the benefits of CST? (Objective 10)

5. As an associate degree graduate, you have been on a medical unit for 15 months. It is your goal to specialize in obstetrics. What steps would you take to begin this process? Would you seek additional formal education? Why or why not? How would you pursue a transfer to the obstetric unit of the hospital? From which professional organization would you seek certification? Provide the rationale for your decision. (Objectives 1 and 2)

6. Your neighbor is an immigrant from Ukraine. In that country she was a nurse, and she asks you how to become a nurse in the United States. What advice would you give to her? (Objectives 5 and 8)

7. You are working as a registered nurse in an ambulatory care setting. A client is very upset about the long wait and the care provided. She states that she thinks this place is "terrible" and that she plans to report everyone. Three weeks later, you receive a letter from the State Board of Nursing informing you that a complaint has been lodged against you for incompetent practice of nursing. Whose advice will you seek? What actions should you take?(Objective 7)

8. In your state, there are legal limitations to licensure associated with chemical dependency and the commission of certain felonies. You had a conviction for driving while under the influence of alcohol when you were 21. At that time you were required to complete an alcohol awareness and education program. You are now 30 years old, graduating from a nursing program and planning to take the licensure examination. The application to take the NCLEX-RN has a list of questions, among them is "Have you ever been treated for an alcohol or chemical dependency related problem? If so, explain." Outline your best course of action. (Objectives 4 and 5)

9. You are interested in becoming certified in critical care nursing. Research the requirements for the CCRN certification offered by the Critical Care Nurses Association. Develop a plan for yourself that could lead to certification. (Objective 9)

10. The hospital in which you work has just announced that it will be increasing the number of unlicensed nursing assistants. From your understanding of the licensure laws in your state, what will be the scope of practice for these unlicensed individuals? (Objective 10)

11. You are working for a long-term care facility. A new person has just joined the Activities/Therapy Department. To work effectively with this person, what information would you need about this person's education and credentials? (Objectives 1 and 2)

## DISCUSSION/ESSAY QUESTIONS

1. Why are credentials for members of health occupations important to the public? (Objective 1)

2. What credentialing mechanisms are used by some allied health professions? (Objective 1)

3. What are the credentials available for nurses? (Objective 1)

4. What is a credential? (Objective 1)

5. Explain the difference between a license and a certificate. (Objective 2)

6. What is certification and what are its advantages as a credentialing method? (Objective 2)

7. Who controls licensure? (Objective 2)

8. Who controls most types of certification? (Objective 2)

9. Anyone who provides health care to the public should be licensed by the state. Agree or disagree with this statement and provide the rationale for your position. (Objectives 2 and 3)

10. Why is a diploma from an accredited school required for licensure? (Objective 2)

11. What are the benefits of mandatory licensure for nursing? (Objective 3)

12. What do you believe to be the most significant event in the history of nursing licensure? Why? (Objective 3)

13. In a situation where mandatory licensure laws exist, what will happen if you practice without a license? (Objective 3)

14. Why did nurses first begin to seek licensure? (Objective 3)

15. Where was the first licensure law enacted? (Objective 3)

16. Which was the first state to have mandatory licensure? (Objective 3)

17. What are the major topics usually included in the Nurse Practice Act? (Objective 4)

18. What is grandfathering in a Nurse Practice Act? (Objective 4)

19. Why do most nurse practice acts contain specific criteria to be used for disciplinary action? (Objective 4)

20. Who controls what is in the Nurse Practice Act itself? (Objective 4)

21. What is meant by a "sunset provision" in a licensing law? (Objective 4)

22. What is "injunctive relief" in a Nurse Practice Act? (Objective 4)

23. Where would the legal definition of nursing be found? (Objective 4)

24. Where would you find the information on the legal scope of practice for the registered nurse? (Objective 4)

25. Describe how rules and regulations are significant to the state law regulating nursing. (Objective 5)

26. What agency is usually charged with administering the Nurse Practice Act? (Objective 5)

27. What is the role of an individual State Board of Nursing in the National Council of State Boards of Nursing? (Objective 5)

28. Why does the State Board of Nursing have the authority to establish rules that affect the practice of nursing? (Objective 5)

29. To whom would you apply for a license as a registered nurse? (Objective 5)

30. What is initial licensure called? (Objective 6)

31. What is licensure in a second jurisdiction called? (Objective 6)

32. If you passed the licensing examination in Texas and want to move to another state, will you need to take the examination again in the new state? (Objective 6)

33. How is the NCLEX-RN examination organized? (Objective 6)

34. What is the minimum number of questions you might take to pass the NCLEX-RN? (Objective 6)

35. What is the organizing pattern for the NCLEX-RN? (Objective 6)

36. Why might you have to meet additional requirements for licensure by endorsement in a new state? (Objective 6)

37. On what grounds might your license as a registered nurse be revoked? (Objective 7)

38. How are graduates of foreign nursing schools admitted to practice in the United States? (Objective 8)

39. What organization evaluates credentials of foreign educated nurses? (Objective 8)

40. If a foreign educated nurse moves to the United States, is he or she automatically eligible to take the NCLEX examination? (Objective 8)

41. What problems are associated with certification in nursing and how might these affect you in the future? (Objective 9)

42. How is certification sometimes related to licensure? (Objective 9)

43. Who controls the requirements for specialty nursing certification? (Objective 9)

44. What is computerized simulation testing? (Objective 10)

45. What is multistate licensure? (Objective 10)

46. How does telenursing relate to multistate licensure? (Objective 10)

## FILL IN THE BLANKS

*Instructions: Complete the following statements by filling in the blanks with the word or words that make the sentence complete and correct.*

1. The two purposes of regulating the practice of any health occupation are to _____ _____ _____ and to _____ _____ _____. (Objective 1)

2. _____ is a process whereby educational institutions are surveyed and evaluated. (Objective 1)

3. The national accreditation of nursing programs is provided by the _____. (Objective 1)

4. Credentials are _____ proof of qualifications. (Objective 1)

5. A license is a _____ _____. (Objective 2)

6. Licensure is controlled by the _____ but certification is usually controlled by _____ _____. (Objective 2)

7. Certification is provided by a _____ authority. (Objective 2)

8. Most organizations actually provide credentialing through an _____ _____. (Objective 2)

9. The organization that originally began the effort to license nurses was the _____ _____ __ _____ __ _____. (Objective 3)

10. _____ licensure is a system whereby an individual may choose to become licensed to provide evidence of competence, but a license is not required to practice. (Objective 3)

11. The first state to pass a mandatory licensure law for registered nurses was _____ _____. (Objective 3)

12. When licensure is required to practice, this is called _____. (Objective 3)

13. In the United States you can expect to find that the licensure law for nursing is _____ rather than permissive. (Objective 3)

14. Some states require completion of _____ _____ to renew a health care license. (Objective 4)

15. The _____ campaigned vigorously for the adoption of state licensure laws. (Objective 3)

16. North Dakota is the first and only state to require a _____ degree for registered nursing. (Objective 4)

17. The organization that originally began the effort to license nurses was the _____ _____ __ ____ _____ _____ _____ _____ (Objective 3)

18. The practice of nursing is legally defined by the _____ _____ ____ _____. (Objective 4)

19. Three common concepts included in the definition of nursing found in nurse practice acts are _____ _____ ____ _____, _____ _____ _____, and _____ _____ _____ _____ _____. (Objective 4)

20. Laws regulating nursing are carried out through _____ and _____. (Objective 4)

21. Model nurse practice acts have been developed by the _____ and the _____. (Objective 4)

22. The Board of Nursing is responsible for developing _____ and _____, which become part of the law. (Objective 5)

23. If you wish to work as an RN in another state, you should contact the _____ _____ ____ _____. (Objective 5)

24. The State Board of Nursing is responsible for _____ _____ against those who have violated the Nurse Practice Act. (Objectives 5 and 7)

25. In most states schools of nursing must be _____ by the State Board of Nursing. (Objective 5)

26. When nurses are concerned whether a particular act falls within the scope of practice allowed by the state, they can request that the Board of Nursing provide an _____ _____. (Objective 5)

27. The members of the board of nursing, in most states, are _____. (Objective 5)

28. The current RN licensure examination is called the _____. (Objective 6)

29. The current nursing licensure examination for practical nursing is called the _____. (Objective 6)

30. Each person taking the examination receives a unique set of questions because the computer program is _____. (Objective 6)

31. The steps of the nursing process as used in the NCLEX-RN are _____, _____, _____, _____, and _____. (Objective 6)

32. The four areas of client needs in the NCLEX-RN examination are _____, _____ _____ _____, _____ _____, _____ _____, and _____ _____. (Objective 6)

33. The process of obtaining a second license in another state is called licensure by_____. (Objective 6)

34. When seeking licensure by endorsement, the applicant_____ _____ all the requirements of the state to which application is being made, if those differ from the requirements of the current state. (Objective 6)

35. A computerized licensure examination that presents different questions to different test takers based on their responses to initial questions is called _____ _____. (Objective 6)

36. Two types of disciplinary action that may be taken by boards of nursing are _____ and _____. (Objective 7)

37. An individual who has violated the Nurse Practice Act is subject to _____ _____ by the State Board of Nursing. (Objective 7)

38. A nurse being investigated for disciplinary action by the Board of Nursing should have the assistance of an _____. (Objective 7)

39. Four common reasons for disciplinary action against a registered nurse are _____, _____, _____, and _____. (Objective 7)

40. Two types of disciplinary action that may be taken by boards of nursing are _____ and _____. (Objective 7)

41. The purposes of the CGFNS examination are to _____ _____ ____ _____ _____ and to _____ _____ _____ ____ ____ _____. (Objective 8)

42. Two organizations that provide certification in a field of nursing are _____ _____ _____ _____ and _____ _____. (Objective 9)

43. The degree most commonly required for certification as a clinical specialist is the _____ _____. (Objective 13)

44. A type of examination being investigated by the NCSBN is computerized _____ testing. (Objective 10)

45. The Pew Commission's recommendations for health professional regulation can be summed up by "SAFE" which stands for _____, _____, _____, _____, and _____. (Objective 10)

## TRUE-FALSE QUESTIONS

*Instructions: Mark the following statements "T" if true or "F" if false. If using a scoring card, mark "A" if true or "B" if false.*

_____ 1. The primary purpose of credentialing health care providers is to protect the public. (Objective 1)

_____ 2. Credentialing guarantees safety for the public. (Objective 1)

_____ 3. One of the strongest reasons for credentialing of health care personnel is for safety of the public. (Objective 1)

_____ 4. The credential that is most actively sought by health care providers is licensure. (Objectives 2 and 3)

_____ 5. Licensure and certification mean the same thing in nursing. (Objective 2)

_____ 6. Interest in establishing nursing licensure began in the 19th century. (Objective 3)

_____ 7. Mandatory licensure means that one must have a license to practice as a registered nurse. (Objective 3)

_____ 8. The state legislative body is responsible for nursing licensure laws. (Objectives 3 and 6)

_____ 9. One of the major goals of the Nurses Associated Alumnae of the United States and Canada was licensure for nurses. (Objective 3)

_____ 10. The first licensure for nurses was introduced in 1865. (Objective 3)

_____ 11. The movement for nursing licensure was begun by Florence Nightingale. (Objective 3)

_____ 12. Nurse practice acts in all states identify the same steps in the nursing process and give them the same name. (Objective 4)

_____ 13. Definitions of practical (vocational) nursing are less restrictive than those for registered nursing. (Objective 4)

_____ 14. Current nursing licensure laws are the same in all states in the United States. (Objectives 4 and 6)

_____ 15. In some states one Nurse Practice Act covers both practical (vocational) nursing and registered nursing. (Objective 4)

_____ 16. Nurse practice acts contain provisions that may allow those who are not licensed to act as nurses in specific situations. (Objective 4)

_____ 17. All changes in the law are grandfathered. (Objective 4)

_____ 18. The State Board of Nursing is free to make any regulations it wishes. (Objective 5)

_____ 19. The Nurse Practice Act spells out the scope of practice. (Objective 5)

_____ 20. The State Board of Nursing must take any disciplinary action to a court for a decision. (Objective 5)

_____ 21. Each State Board of Nursing is elected by the citizens of that state. (Objective 5)

_____ 22. The NCLEX-RN examination is based on research that identifies the essential safe behavior of the beginning nurse. (Objective 8)

_____ 23. Once one has obtained a nursing license in any state, it will never be necessary to take the basic licensing examination again. (Objective 6)

_____ 24. All states require a passing score on a comprehensive examination but do not name the examination in the law. (Objective 6)

_____ 25. In some states license renewal requires only payment of a fee. (Objective 6)

_____ 21. All applicants seeking licensure as a practical or registered nurse should participate in a formal review course. (Objective 6)

_____ 27. Computerized examinations began in 1992 in all states. (Objective 6)

_____ 28. Conviction of a drug-related crime is a reason for revocation of a nursing license in most states. (Objective 7)

_____ 29. Disciplinary action by a State Board of Nursing always results in loss of a license to practice nursing. (Objective 7)

_____ 30. If a nurse believes that he or she has acted correctly and not violated the Nurse Practice Act, it is not necessary to have an attorney in a disciplinary proceeding. (Objective 7)

_____ 31. Chemical dependency will always result in immediate revocation of a license to practice nursing. (Objective 7)

_____ 32. A consumer can report an individual to the Board of Nursing for substandard practice. (Objective 7)

_____ 33. Graduates of foreign nursing schools MUST take the CGFNS examination in their own countries before coming to the United States. (Objective 8)

_____ 34. Nursing licenses can be transferred internationally through the International Congress of Nursing. (Objective 8)

_____ 35. Nursing education differs greatly from country to country. (Objective 8)

_____ 36. All certification for nurse practitioners requires a master's degree. (Objective 9)

_____ 37. All nursing organizations are united in providing certification through a single credentialing center. (Objective 9)

_____ 38. Some certifications are recognized by State Boards of Nursing as meeting a legal standard for advanced practice in nursing. (Objective 9)

_____ 39. All nurse anesthetists are certificated by the Council on Certification of Nurse Anesthetists. (Objective 9)

_____ 40. Titles for nurses in advanced practice are now standardized throughout the United States. (Objective 9)

_____ 41. Computerized simulation testing (CST) will become a part of the NCLEX-RN examination in 2002. (Objective 10)

_____ 42. The Pew Commission made the recommendation that the principles of SAFE (Standardized, Accountable, Flexible, Effective, and Efficient) be applied to health professional licensure. (Objective 10)

_____ 43. A major concern in the future will be ensuring continuing competency of health professionals who are already licensed. (Objective 10)

## MATCHING QUESTIONS

*Instructions: Match the numbered items with the most appropriate lettered items.*

### Group A (Objective 2)

_____ 1. Permissive licensure

_____ 2. Mandatory licensure

_____ 3. Certification

_____ 4. Credentials

_____ 5. Diploma

    a. Any official document that attests to one's status or abilities.

    b. A system that provides for legal recognition of those in a profession who wish to have it.

    c. A system that requires those in a profession to have legal recognition of their qualifications.

    d. A method by which a profession identifies ability and attests to a person's qualifications to practice.

    e. A written certificate attesting to educational attainment.

### Group B (Objective 2)

_____ 1. Accreditation

_____ 2. Certificate

_____ 3. Credential

_____ 4. Diploma/degree

_____ 5. License

    a. Written proof of one's qualifications to carry out specific activities.

    b. Usually granted on completion of an educational program and the passing of a standardized examination.

    c. Usually recognizes completion of a designated program of study such as high school.

    d. A legal credential.

    e. Status awarded to an organization when specified standards have been met.

## MULTIPLE-CHOICE QUESTIONS

*Instructions: Choose the one best answer for each question.*

1. Which of the following is true regarding the concept of credentialing?

    a. Credentials are written proof of qualifications.

    b. Credentials always provide legal verification of competence to practice.

    c. There are but a few types of credentials.

    d. Credentials are awarded only by the State Board of Nursing.

    (Objective 1)

2. Which of the following are professionals who are licensed in all states?

    a. Physicians, psychologists, pharmacists, and nurses

    b. Psychologists, pharmacists, dentists, and nurses

    c. Physicians, dentists, psychologists, and nurses

    d. Physicians, dentists, pharmacists, and nurses

    (Objective 1)

3. Which of the following statements is true of the credentialing of health occupations?

    a. Most health occupations are now credentialed through a national voluntary system.

    b. There are national criteria that states use to determine whether or not a given occupation should be licensed.

c. Each state has acted independently on which (if any) health occupations must be credentialed.

d. All health occupations are required to demonstrate competence through continuing education.

(Objective 1)

4. What is one of the arguments against having professional groups accredit programs in their own area of expertise?

a. Loss of objectivity

b. Cost

c. Lack of skilled accreditors

d. Lack of standards

(Objectives 1, 2)

5. How does licensing differ from certification?

a. It is not revocable.

b. It is more costly.

c. It confers a legal status.

d. It is recognized nationally in all health professions.

(Objective 2)

6. What is one of the methods through which specialized preparation is recognized in health care?

a. Certification

b. Accreditation

c. Verification

d. Validation

(Objective 2)

7. Who usually grants certification?

a. State agency

b. Professional organization

c. Employing institution

d. None of the above

(Objective 2)

8. Who grants a diploma?

a. State agency

b. Professional organization

c. Employing institution

d. Anyone who provides an educational program

(Objective 2)

9. Who grants a license to practice?

a. State agency

b. Professional organization

c. Employing institution

d. College or university

(Objective 2)

10. Which factor contributed most to uniformity of standards for registration of nurses throughout the United States?

a. The pressure of the public for uniformity

b. Federal legislation

c. National accreditation of schools

d. Demands of hospitals for adequately prepared nurses

(Objective 2)

11. Which of the following is a requirement of mandatory licensure?

a. Meeting the established standards

b. Graduating from an accredited program

c. Being of legally responsible age

d. Listing one's name and credentials with a registry

(Objective 3)

12. What do nurses who oppose permissive rather than mandatory licensure believe?

    a. It will be more difficult to keep track of where nurses are employed.

    b. The state will lose revenue from licensure fees.

    c. Patients may be jeopardized by potentially lower quality care.

    d. It could result in a shortage of nurses.

    (Objective 3)

13. What is a license law that permits nurses either to practice without a license or obtain a license?

    a. Compulsory

    b. Comprehensive

    c. Permissive

    d. Mandatory

    (Objective 3)

14. Which was the first state to enact mandatory licensure for registered nurses?

    a. Washington

    b. Ohio

    c. New York

    d. Illinois

    (Objective 3)

15. If you are licensed in one state and move to another, what must you do?

    a. Simply notify the new state of your current license in order to practice

    b. Apply to retake the licensing examination

    c. Pay a fee to be immediately granted a license by reciprocity

    d. Meet all the requirements for licensure of the new state

    (Objective 3)

16. Which of the following is the legal guide to the practice of registered nursing?

    a. ANA Code of Ethics

    b. Nightingale Pledge

    c. State practice act

    d. Patient's Bill of Rights

    (Objective 4)

17. Which of the following describes the definitions of nursing included in laws regulating nursing practice?

    a. They differentiate between baccalaureate and associate degree practice.

    b. They define the scope of practice.

    c. They support master's preparation for beginning practice.

    d. They mandate continuing education.

    (Objective 4)

18. Major content areas in laws regulating nursing practice include purpose, definitions, and which of the following?

    a. Licensure fees

    b. Role of the medical examining committee

    c. Listing of approved schools

    d. Qualifications for licensure

    (Objective 4)

19. What is a provision in a revised nurse practice that allows current RNs to continue in practice even if they do not meet the new standard?

    a. Grandfather clause

    b. Maintenance of license clause

    c. Retention clause

    d. Continuation clause

    (Objective 4)

20. Which of the following definitions of nursing will most affect your practice?

    a. The one used by the ANA.

    b. The one developed by the nursing theorist you choose to follow.

c. The one found in the Nurse Practice Act.

d. The one adopted by the facility or agency for which you work.

(Objective 4)

21. The role of the Board of Nursing includes establishing standards for licensure, enforcing disciplinary codes, regulating specialty practice, and which of the following?

    a. Approving nursing education programs

    b. Determining sites for education programs

    c. Approving master's and doctoral programs in nursing

    d. Establishing working conditions for nurses employed in hospital settings

    (Objective 5)

22. What is the common responsibility of the State Board of Nursing as established by the licensure laws?

    a. Establish essential content for curricula in nursing schools

    b. License health care institutions

    c. Negotiate nurses' salaries

    d. Write the licensing examination

    (Objective 5)

23. What is a common responsibility of the State Board of Nursing identified in the Nurse Practice Act?

    a. Set standards for nursing care

    b. Discipline individuals who have violated provisions of the Nurse Practice Act

    c. Choose future members of the board

    d. Provide specialty certification

    (Objective 5)

24. Which of the following is true regarding nursing licensure?

    a. It is active throughout a lifetime.

b. It can be revoked under certain circumstances.

c. It requires retaking the examination if you move from one state to another.

d. It requires that all applicants be high school graduates.

(Objectives 4, 5, and 7)

25. If you were licensed in Iowa and wished to accept a nursing position in Chicago, Illinois, you would need to do which of the following?

    a. Practice using the Iowa license

    b. Apply to the state of Illinois to take the Illinois licensing examination

    c. Apply to the state of Illinois for interstate endorsement

    d. Apply to the state of Iowa for transfer of your license to Illinois

    (Objective 8)

26. The common state requirements for licensure as a registered nurse include which of the following?

    a. United States citizenship

    b. Graduation from an NLN-accredited school

    c. Baccalaureate degree

    d. Passing score on the licensure examination

    (Objective 6)

27. What is the purpose of the licensing examination?

    a. Differentiate levels of excellence

    b. Demonstrate basic safe practice

    c. Establish information to be used for admission to graduate school

    d. Screen and limit the number of registered nurses

    (Objective 6)

28. Which of the following is true regarding computerized adapted testing?

    a. Candidates know immediately whether they have passed or failed.

    b. It presents the same questions to all candidates.

    c. It presents the same questions in a situation format.

    d. It evaluates each response and then selects an appropriate question to present next.

    (Objective 6)

29. The role of the Commission on Graduates of Foreign Nursing Schools (CGFNS) includes which of the following?

    a. Establishing fees for foreign graduates

    b. Assisting foreign graduates with English comprehension

    c. Preparing foreign graduates to take the NCLEX for registered nursing

    d. Investigating and validating credentials held by graduates of foreign nursing schools

    (Objective 8)

30. Which of the following statements is true of certification?

    a. Certification is a type of credentialing that has professional status.

    b. Certification is a type of credentialing that has legal status.

    c. Certification is available only through the ANA.

    d. Certification must always be endorsed by the Board of Nursing.

    (Objective 9)

31. What process is generally used to recognize specialty training and education in nursing?

    a. Licensure

    b. Certification

    c. Accreditation

    d. Documentation

    (Objective 9)

32. All certification represents which of the following?

    a. Postbaccalaureate preparation

    b. Master's degree preparation

    c. Completion of program of study

    d. Completion of a home study course

    (Objective 9)

33. Which of the following statements is true of certification?

    a. All state nursing practice acts recognize certification as a standard for specialty practice.

    b. All hospitals use specialty certification for purposes of establishing salaries and giving promotions.

    c. Certification is understood by the public to represent excellence in practice.

    d. Certification requires that the applicant meet predetermined standards for specialty practice.

    (Objective 9)

34. Which of the following was the major recommendation of the Study of Credentialing in Nursing?

    a. Eliminate specialized certification

    b. Establish an independent, free-standing center for nursing credentialing

    c. Turn all credentialing over to the professional associations

    d. Move toward institutional licensure

    (Objective 10)

35. What was the immediate effect of the recommendation of the Study of Credentialing on the credentialing

process in nursing?

a. Credentialing has been moved to the state boards of nursing.

b. Credentialing is gradually being consolidated under a free-standing credentialing center.

c. Credentialing is being coordinated by the professional association of nurses.

d. Study and discussion are continuing.

(Objective 9)

36. Which of the following may be a future trend in nursing licensure?

a. Computerized adapted testing

b. Computerized simulated testing

c. Paper/pencil testing

d. Oral examinations

(Objective 10)

# GAMING IN THE CLASSROOM

*Instructions: This game involves selecting teams and a host. The teams compete against one another for points. Each game has several subject categories. After teams are determined, a team is chosen to go first and selects a category. The host then poses the answer and the team provides the correct question for that answer. Each question can be awarded the same number of points or more difficult questions may be given heavier point values. (The instructor might determine which questions are more difficult based on the content emphasized in class.) Points are awarded to the team that is the first to signal and give a correct question. If that team is incorrect, the other team may attempt to provide the correct question and receive the points. The length of time allowed for response can be determined by the class or by the instructor. The team with the most points at the end of the game is declared the winner. Teams may be composed of individual students or groups of students. Teams may determine their answers as a team or may take turns answering as individuals.*

## Categories

A. Differentiating Credentials

B. History of Nursing Licensure

C. Topics within Nursing Practice Act

D. Role of the State Board of Nursing

## Answers and Questions

### Category A

A:  License.

Q:  What is the legal credential called?

A:  Certificate.

Q:  What type of credential identifies specialty practice?

A:  Diploma.

Q:  What type of credential identifies educational accomplishment?

A:  Accreditation.

Q:  What type of credential attests to the quality of an educational program?

### Category B

A:  North Carolina.

Q:  What was the first state to institute nursing licensure?

A:  New York.

Q:  What was the first state to institute mandatory nursing licensure?

A:  Graduate nurse.

Q:  What was the title used by those who had not met the standard for permissive licensure?

A:  Nurses Associated Alumni of the United States and Canada.

Q:  What was the first organization to promote nursing licensure?

A:  1923.

Q:  What was the year when all states had enacted permissive licensure laws?

## Category C

A: Protection of the public.

Q: What is the primary purpose of licensure laws?

A: Directed scope of nursing practice.

Q: What is a common definition of practical nursing?

A: Passing score on the NCLEX-RN.

Q: What is a requirement for licensure in all states?

A: Grandfather clause.

Q: What provision of the law protects the practice of those currently licensed when changes are made in the requirements for licensure?

A: Continuing education.

Q: What is a requirement for licensure renewal in many states?

## Category D

A: Monitoring program.

Q: What is one type of disciplinary action that can be taken by the State Board of Nursing?

A: Appointment by the governor.

Q: How are most members of Boards of Nursing chosen?

A: Provide for interstate endorsement.

Q: What is the Board of Nursing role in relationship to registered nurses moving from other states?

A: Revocation of license.

Q: What is the most severe penalty the Board of Nursing can apply?

A: National Council of State Boards of Nursing.

Q: What is the organization made up of State Boards of Nursing?

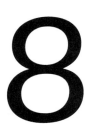

# Legal Responsibilities for Practice

## PURPOSE

This chapter provides a basic foundation for understanding how the law regulates the practice of nursing. The sources of law and how law is administered are explained to enhance the student's understanding of negligence, malpractice, and liability. Specific situations and legal cases pertinent to liability are presented along with suggestions for preventing legal actions.

## OBJECTIVES

1. Identify two general sources of law and describe their differences.

2. Explain the role of institutional policies and protocols in legal decision making.

3. Describe some situations in which nurses may be involved in criminal law.

4. Define liability, identifying situations in which liability is shared by employers or supervisors.

5. State points to be considered in the purchase of professional liability insurance.

6. List the most commonly recurring legal issues in nursing.

7. Explain how informed consent, advance directives, and the Patient Self-Determination Act support the patient's rights.

8. Discuss the nurse's responsibility in the specific issues that can constitute malpractice.

9. Identify factors that contribute to a suit being instituted against a health care professional and how an individual nurse might prevent legal suits.

10. Explain the various aspects of testifying for a legal proceeding.

## KEY TERMS

Administrative law
Advance directive
Claims brought insurance
Claims occurred insurance
Common law
Court
Criminal law
Deposition
Discovery
Durable power of attorney
Durable power of attorney for health care
Guardian
Informed consent
Liability
Liability insurance
Malpractice
Minor
Negligence
Patient Self-Determination Act
Privileged communication
Regulatory law
Res ipsa loquitor
Statutory law
Suit
Testimony
Tort

## SITUATIONS TO FOSTER CRITICAL THINKING

1. Explain what is meant by the statement "Your professional responsibilities rest on a dual framework of legal and ethical constraints." How do ethics influence our professional practice? Give an example of an instance in which ethics affect our actions as nurses. Give an example of an instance in which our actions are affected by both ethical and legal considerations. Give an example of a situation having both ethical and legal concerns in which the two are divergent. (Objective 1)

2. You have been working for 6 months in a small community hospital that has very limited visiting hours—2–4 P.M. and 7–9 P.M. You believe that the patients would respond better to a more liberal visitation policy. You do not believe, as do some of the nurses and physicians, that this is disruptive to the care routine. How would you go about seeking a change in this policy? What group within the hospital develops the policy? Who enforces it? What strategies might be used to make the change? (Objective 2)

3. As a nurse with 2 years of experience, you have just obtained the position in intensive care that was your goal. However, the situation is much different than you had imagined. Many of your patients do not survive, and you believe that you are often contributing to prolonging death rather than preserving life. One concern you have is the lack of any clear guidelines for dealing with end-of-life issues. What information about advance directives, informed consent, and the Patient Self-Determination Act is relevant to your concerns? How might you begin to affect policies in your institution in regard to these issues? (Objectives 2 and 7)

4. A family member of one of the patients on the unit where you work nights has complained to the administration that a large sum of money and a valuable ring were stolen from the patient's bedside stand sometime in the last 24 hours. The family member has called police to report the crime and demanded that the hospital find the criminal. Your supervisor decides to interview everyone who worked on that unit during the last 24 hours. You do remember that it was a very busy night because you had admitted a person after an auto accident. There were family members, transport assistants, laboratory personnel, and others on the unit in addition to the regular staff. What concerns might you have about this situation? What is your legal obligation to the patient and to the hospital? (Objective 3)

5. In your new position as a registered nurse in a nursing home, you are responsible for supervising two licensed practical nurses who give all medications and do treatments, and six to eight nursing assistants who provide personal care. If one of the LPNs makes a serious medication error, what is your exposure to liability? If one of the nursing assistants forgets a safety device and a resident falls, what is your exposure to liability? What could you do to minimize your risks of liability problems in this setting? (Objective 4)

6. You have just received your license to practice as a registered nurse and are employed on the evening shift in a skilled nursing facility. Occasionally you are the charge nurse for that shift. Today's mail included an unsolicited letter offering you the opportunity to purchase personal liability insurance through your state nurses association for $67 per year. How will you respond to this offer? What information will you need to make a decision? Where will you obtain that information? Why did you respond as you did? (Objective 5)

7. You have just accepted a job in a psychiatric hospital that cares for both involuntarily committed patients and voluntary patients. What issues of false imprisonment are a concern in this environment? Where will you go to find out how to manage these issues? (Objective 6)

8. John Miles, a next-door neighbor, recently suffered a cardiovascular accident and is now making a slow but positive recovery. However, his wife has been concerned about advance directives as a result of their recent experiences. She has asked you for information on advance directives. Assuming that she knows almost nothing, what information would you provide? What resources would you suggest she contact? What are your legal constraints, if any, in providing this information? Would it be appropriate for you to witness any legal documents that are signed? (Objectives 7, 8, and 9)

9. You have been asked by a neighbor whether the physician they have chosen as a pediatrician is a good one. You have worked with this pediatrician and have not been favorably impressed by his approach to families. It seems to you that families receive limited teaching; their questions are quickly brushed off; and they are asked to make decisions without being given time and support. What legal issues does this present to you? How might you respond both legally and ethically to this challenge? (Objective 8)

10. You are working in a nursing home and one of your responsibilities is maintaining the care plans for the residents on your unit. This responsibility is shared with all nurses who work on that unit during the various shifts and days of the week. A resident who is receiving Coumadin daily and a PT test weekly, develops grossly bloody urine. She is transferred to a hospital where she dies in renal failure due to bleeding in the kidneys. Her family is suing the nursing home for not identifying this problem sooner. You were not working when the bleeding was noted. What might affect your liability for a malpractice claim in this situation? (Objective 8)

11. As a nurse working in a home care agency, how will you incorporate the expectations regarding patient self-determination into your practice? (Objective 8)

12. You have been asked by your head nurse to prepare a presentation to be shared with other employees on your unit regarding actions nurses can take to prevent the initiation of lawsuits. What would be the most important points you would want to emphasize in the presentation? What resources or resource persons would you contact in your facility? What organizations might you want to contact for information? Where would you begin? (Objectives 6, 8, and 9)

13. You are employed as a staff nurse on a telemetry unit. Three months ago a patient on the unit suffered a cardiac arrest after falling from her bed. The family has brought a lawsuit against the hospital, claiming negligence. Although you did not care for the patient, you have received a subpoena to give testimony in the form of a deposition regarding unit protocol. What information do you need? From whom will you obtain that information? When giving your deposition what should you keep in mind? Where will you likely give the deposition? Who can you expect to find in attendance? (Objectives 2, 8, and 10)

## DISCUSSION/ESSAY QUESTIONS

1. What is the difference between common law and statutory law? (Objective 1)

2. What is the difference between enacted law and regulatory law? (Objective 1)

3. Who has authority and responsibility for changing enacted law? (Objective 1)

4. Give an example of enacted law. (Objective 1)

5. Give an example of regulatory law. (Objective 1)

6. Give an example of how civil law affects nurses. (Objective 1)

7. Give an example of how criminal law affects nurses. (Objective 1)

8. What is a major source of common law in health care facilities or agencies? (Objective 2)

9. What are sources of standards of nursing practice that might be construed as representing common law? (Objective 2)

10. How might a court use institutional policy in making a decision about the liability of a nurse in a lawsuit for malpractice? (Objective 2)

11. Give an example of how a nurse might be involved in criminal law. (Objective 3)

12. Breaking laws regarding controlled substances is a violation of what kind of law? (Objective 3)

13. If you observe someone in a health care facility engaging in what you believe to be a criminal act (such as falsifying a narcotic record), what is your responsibility? (Objective 3)

14. If a "minor" criminal act by a nurse is not prosecuted by the authorities, what other consequences might there be? (Objective 3)

15. What constitutes a "crime"? (Objective 3)

16. What is liability? (Objective 4)

17. Give an example of how a supervisor or charge nurse might share liability with a staff member. (Objective 4)

18. What is meant by "respondeat superior"? (Objective 4)

19. Explain how an institution can be held liable for the actions of employees. (Objective 4)

20. When an individual is found liable for an adverse outcome, what is the usual remedy awarded by the court? (Objective 4)

21. What is the difference between a liability insurance policy that provides coverage for claims made during the life of the policy and one that provides coverage for incidents that occurred during the life of the policy? (Objective 5)

22. What are differences between coverage by an employer's liability policy and coverage by a personal liability policy? (Objective 5)

23. Give two situations in which you would not be covered by an employer's liability policy. (Objective 5)

24. What is meant by defamation of character, and how might a  nurse be involved in a legal action with regard to this issue? (Objective 6)

25. In which situations might false imprisonment be a concern for nurses? (Objective 6)

26. What constitutes fraud in the practice of nursing? (Objective 6)

27. List three instances in which a nurse might have privileged information. (Objective 6)

28. What are the potential concerns regarding confidentiality when records are computerized? (Objective 6)

29. When can a patient legally be prevented from leaving a health care facility? (Objective 6)

30. Describe a situation in which the nurse is responsible for obtaining informed consent. (Objective 7)

31. What does the Patient Self-Determination Act require? (Objective 7)

32. What is an advance directive? (Objective 7)

33. What is a durable power of attorney for health care? (Objective 7)

34. What is a power of attorney? (Objective 7)

35. What is a living will? (Objective 7)

36. What is the difference between a living will and a durable power of attorney for health care? (Objective 7)

37. How is malpractice different from negligence? (Objective 8)

38. What is meant by the term *reasonably prudent nurse*? (Objective 8)

39. When does a nurse have a legal "duty" toward another individual? (Objective 8)

40. How might a court use the concept of a reasonably prudent nurse in making a decision relative to the liability of a nurse in a lawsuit for malpractice? (Objectives 1 and 8)

41. In which situations might defamation of character be a concern for nurses? (Objective 8)

42. Discuss actions a nurse could take to prevent a lawsuit. (Objective 9)

43. What factors might identify a suit-prone patient? (Objective 9)

44. Why is it prudent to have legal counsel before giving a deposition? (Objective 10)

45. What resources are available for you to consult before testifying in a legal action? (Objective 10)

46. What should you do if, when testifying, you are asked a question about something you do not remember? (Objective 10)

47. If you are testifying and have to go to the bathroom, what should you do? (Objective 10)

## FILL IN THE BLANKS

*Instructions: Complete the following statements by filling in the blanks with the word or words that make the sentence complete and correct.*

1. Principles of conduct governing one's relationship with others are known as _____. (Objective 1)

2. _____ includes those rules of conduct or action recognized as binding or enforced by a controlling authority such as local, state, or national government. (Objective 1)

3. Law enacted by a legislative body is _____ law. (Objective 1)

4. Enacted laws and regulatory laws fall in the category of _____ law. (Objective 1)

5. Laws relating to crimes against society as a whole make up the body of _____ law. (Objective 1)

6. Law derived from common usage, custom, and judicial decisions or court rulings is known as _____ law. (Objective 1)

7. Laws relating to problems between individuals or businesses that do not affect society as a whole make up the body of _____ law. (Objective 1)

8. A violation of civil law is termed a _____. (Objective 1)

9. A violation of criminal law is termed a _____. (Objective 1)

10. Law derived from usual practice, such as that seen in policy manuals, is called _____ law. (Objective 2)

11. If you needed to decide who could give consent in a particular situation in a hospital, you would first seek this information from a _____ _____. (Objective 2)

12. If an attorney was reviewing care in a specific case, she might look in a _____ _____ to determine what actions the nurse should have taken in the situation. (Objective 2)

13. If the nurse becomes aware that someone else in the health care environment has committed a crime, the nurse is required to _____ it. (Objective 3)

14. Fraud in maintaining narcotic records could be prosecuted as a _____. (Objective 3)

15. Making an error that resulted in harm to a patient would be tried under _____ law. (Objective 3)

16. In addition to criminal prosecution, the licensed person committing a crime in a health care environment might also lose _____. (Objective 3)

17. If the nurse observed an assault on a nursing home resident, the nurse would be expected to report this situation to _____ _____. (Objective 3)

18. The instance in which the employer can be held responsible for the torts committed by an employee is known as _____ _____. (Objective 4)

19. When a nonprofit hospital cannot be held legally liable for harm done to a patient by its employees, it is said to have _____ _____.
(Objective 4)

20. The organization that charitable immunity exempts from liability is _____. (Objective 4)

21. If you are the charge nurse, a key aspect of protecting yourself against liability for acts committed by those you supervise is _____ appropriately. (Objective 4)

22. Insurance that covers incidents that occurred while the policy was in force, regardless of when the claim is brought, is known as _____ _____. (Objective 5)

23. Insurance that covers incidents only if the claim is made while the policy is currently in force is known as _____ _____. (Objective 5)

24. _____ _____ transfers the costs of being sued and of any settlement from the individual to a large group. (Objective 5)

25. Liability insurance of your employer would *not* cover your actions when you were a _____. (Objective 5)

26. Any time that shared information is detrimental to the person's reputation, the person sharing the information may be liable for _____ __ _____. (Objective 6)

27. Using restraints to confine a person against his or her will is called _____ _____. (Objective 6)

28. A family member asks to see a patient's record. Allowing this would be a breach of _____. (Objective 6)

29. To give effective consent, the individual must be _____. (Objective 7)

30. To be acceptable in a court, consent must be both _____ and _____. (Objective 7)

31. If a person is determined to be incompetent, consent is given by the _____ _____. (Objective 7)

32. Causing injury by failure to behave as a reasonably prudent person is _____. (Objective 8)

33. Proving malpractice requires that the following four points be demonstrated: _____, _____, _____ ___ _____, and _____ _____ _____ _____ _____ _____ _____ _____. (Objective 8)

34. Causing injury to a person for whom one is responsible by failing to behave as a reasonably prudent professional is _____. (Objective 8)

35. One characteristic of the suit-prone patient is that he or she may often be _____. (Objective 9)

36. One action a nurse might take to prevent the initiation of a suit is to _____ _____ _____ _____. (Objective 9)

37. A written legal testimony is called a (an) _____. (Objective 10)

38. The process of seeking information regarding a possible legal action is termed _____. (Objective 10)

39. _____ refers to information shared with certain professionals that does not need to be revealed even in a court of law. (Objective 10)

40. If you have special knowledge and expertise in an area of nursing, you might be asked to testify as an _____ witness. (Objective 10)

# TRUE-FALSE QUESTIONS

*Instructions: Mark the following statements "T" if true or "F" if false. If using a scoring card, mark "A" if true or "B" if false.*

_____ 1. Statutory law is the same as enacted law. (Objective 1)

_____ 2. Crimes occurring in health care settings are always prosecuted. (Objective 1)

_____ 3. Common law includes judicial decisions. (Objective 1)

_____ 4. Rules and regulations of a governmental administrative body are considered law. (Objective 1)

_____ 5. A violation of civil law is termed a tort. (Objective 1)

_____ 6. Rules and regulations for nursing are enacted by the various state legislatures. (Objective 1)

_____ 7. Statutory law derives from common usage, custom, and judicial decisions or court rulings. (Objective 1)

_____ 8. A violation of civil law can be punished by a jail term. (Objective 1)

_____ 9. Institutional policy is not relevant to a discussion of legal liability. (Objective 2)

_____ 10. If you follow an institutional policy, you are protected from liability even if the policy is outdated and erroneous. (Objective 2)

_____ 11. A protocol might be considered by a court to represent common law. (Objective 2)

_____ 12. Falsifying a narcotic record is a crime. (Objective 3)

_____ 13. All crimes that occur in a nursing home are prosecuted by the authorities. (Objective 3)

_____ 14. If a nurse knows that a crime has occurred in his or her place of employment, the nurse should avoid involvement with the situation. (Objective 3)

_____ 15. If a nurse fails to report a crime, the nurse may be subject to loss of a license to practice. (Objective 3)

_____ 16. The standard of the reasonably prudent nurse applies to the student nurse. (Objective 4)

_____ 17. Liability means that one is legally responsible for what occurs. (Objective 4)

_____ 18. A supervisor is always responsible when an employee is negligent. (Objective 4)

_____ 19. If you carry out your supervisory responsibilities correctly, you may avoid liability for errors of those you supervise. (Objective 4)

_____ 20. Licensed individuals have more responsibility independent of the supervisor or employer than do unlicensed individuals. (Objective 4)

_____ 21. Nurses do not need to purchase professional liability insurance because no one sues a person who has no insurance. (Objective 5)

_____ 22. If you had any type of malpractice liability insurance when an incident occurred, you can be sure that you will be covered even if the suit is brought years later. (Objective 5)

_____ 23. An employer's liability insurance coverage will not cover you when you are acting in a volunteer capacity. (Objective 5)

_____ 24. An employer's liability insurance coverage will cover you if you stop at an auto accident on the way to work. (Objective 5)

_____ 25. It is possible for a nurse who restrains a patient in a bed without a medical order to be charged with false imprisonment. (Objective 6)

_____ 26. Res ipsa loquitor refers to a legal ruling that a situation speaks for itself and does not need further proof. (Objective 6)

_____ 27. When faxing patient information from a hospital to a home care agency, you do not have to worry about confidentiality. (Objective 6)

_____ 28. A nurse is never liable for anything that relates to medical care. (Objective 6)

_____ 29. A minor can never give consent. (Objective 7)

_____ 30. Some states recognize the category of emancipated minor. (Objective 7)

_____ 31. A person can be competent to make some informed decisions but considered incompetent to make others. (Objective 7)

_____ 32. Every facility or agency that receives Medicare or Medicaid money is required by law to inform patients that they have the right to self-determination and can establish advance directives. (Objective 7)

_____ 33. In an emergency situation, consent is often implied. (Objective 7)

_____ 34. *Malpractice* is a term used for a specific type negligence. (Objective 8)

_____ 35. If you do not have a duty to a person, you cannot be liable. (Objective 8)

_____ 36. If no harm occurs, there is no malpractice. (Objective 8)

_____ 37. If a person does not have physical harm, there is no malpractice. (Objective 8)

_____ 38. Patients who constantly find fault and criticize care are rarely the individuals who file lawsuits. (Objective 9)

_____ 39. There is nothing one can do to prevent malpractice suits. (Objective 9)

_____ 40. A deposition requires the same standard of truthfulness as required when one is testifying in court. (Objective 10)

_____ 41. It is not legal for a nurse to provide a court with information regarding a conversation with a patient. (Objective 10)

## MATCHING QUESTIONS

*Instructions: Match the numbered items with the most appropriate lettered items.*

### Group A (Objective 6)

_____ 1. Fraud

_____ 2. False imprisonment

_____ 3. Battery

_____ 4. Assault

_____ 5. Slander

_____ 6. Libel

a. Oral defamation of character

b. Written defamation of character

c. Refusing to allow a person to leave a hospital

d. Threatening to touch a person in an unwanted manner

e. Touching a person in an unwanted manner

f. Deliberate deception for personal gain

## MULTIPLE-CHOICE QUESTIONS

*Instructions: Choose the one best answer for each question.*

1. Statutory law consists of two categories. One contains those laws enacted by legislative bodies such as a city council or state legislature. The other includes rules and regulations established by which of the following?

a. Congress

b. Governmental agencies such as licensing boards

c. Supreme Court

d. Local municipalities

(Objective 1)

2. Which of the following is one of the two general sources of law?

    a. Criminal law

    b. Community law

    c. Statutory law

    d. Constitutional law

    (Objective 1)

3. What is our common law derived from?

    a. Laws enacted by legislative bodies

    b. Laws established by governmental agencies

    c. Laws that regulate conduct between private individuals

    d. Usage, custom, and judicial decisions

    (Objective 1)

4. What does civil law consist of?

    a. Laws that affect the public welfare as a whole

    b. Laws that regulate conduct between private individuals or businesses

    c. Laws generated from common usage and custom

    d. Laws enacted by legislative bodies

    (Objective 1)

5. What is the major purpose of institutional policies?

    a. To serve as guidelines to protect the institution and its employees from legal difficulties

    b. To form the basis for performance evaluation of employees

    c. To meet Joint Commission on Accreditation of Healthcare Organization standards

    d. To establish in writing the hospital's organizational hierarchy

    (Objective 2)

6. If an institutional policy does not reflect the best current practice, what should you do?

    a. Follow the policy because that is always common law.

    b. Do not follow the policy but use your best judgment.

    c. Seek to change the policy.

    d. Report the problem to your supervisor and ask the supervisor to make all decisions.

    (Objective 2)

7. What is the major purpose of institutional policy?

    a. To protect individual employees from difficulties

    b. To protect patients from errors

    c. To limit the potential for liability of the institution

    d. To provide a legal defense in case of a lawsuit.

    (Objective 2)

8. Why might institutional policy be presented in a court of law?

    a. It is always considered the correct action.

    b. It is an indicator of standard practice.

    c. It must be considered as common law.

    d. It will be of interest to jurors.

    (Objective 2)

9. What is the correct action if a nurse observes what might a be considered evidence of child abuse?

    a. In most jurisdictions the nurse would be prohibited from reporting this because of laws relating to confidentiality.

    b. If a client told the nurse anything about what happened, the nurse cannot report it because of client-nurse privilege.

c. The nurse should use professional judgment in regard to what would work out best for the child.

d. In most jurisdictions the nurse is required to report to authorities any evidence of child abuse.

(Objective 3)

10. A physician orders a very large dose of intravenous narcotic for a terminally ill patient. The nurse believes this will cause the patient to die. Legally, the nurse

a. cannot be prosecuted for a crime if the doctor ordered the medication.

b. is responsible for any medication he or she gives.

c. can give the medication if it is approved by the supervisor.

d. should notify the authorities immediately.

(Objective 3)

11. If the nurse changes a medication record to avoid having to search for a missing narcotic dose, what would this be treated as?

a. A crime

b. A tort

c. Negligence

d. Malpractice

(Objective 3)

12. When is an act usually considered a crime?

a. When it affects another individual monetarily

b. When it affects the general welfare of the public

c. When it is related to conduct between private individuals or businesses

d. When it is very serious

(Objective 3)

13. What is the legal term that indicates that an employer has responsibility for the actions of its employees?

a. Respondeat superior

b. Res ipsa loquitor

c. Summa cum laude

d. Gaudeamus igitur

(Objective 4)

14. In which situation would a charge nurse be legally liable for the action of a member of the staff whom he or she had assigned for the day?

a. When the staff member makes any error

b. When the staff member makes an error that relates to patient safety issues

c. When the staff member has been assigned to a task that is not within his or her training

d. When a staff member fails to report to the charge nurse

(Objective 4)

15. What is referred to as being legally responsible for the outcome of an action?

a. Liability

b. Responsibility

c. Intentional tort

d. Negligence

(Objective 4)

16. Could assets held by you and your spouse jointly be claimed by an individual receiving a judgment against you in a malpractice suit?

a. Not under any circumstances

b. Yes, in certain states

c. Only if you are head of a household

d. Only if you own at least 51% of the assets

(Objective 4)

17. If you assign tasks to a nursing assistant, are you legally liable for whether those tasks were done correctly?

    a. Never.

    b. Not usually, if the tasks are within the scope of the nursing assistant's training and job description.

    c. Always, that is part of being a supervisor.

    d. Situations vary so much that you would need legal advice on each individual situation.

    (Objective 4)

18. What is a policy that covers a claim whether or not you currently have coverage?

    a. Claims brought policy

    b. Claims occurred policy

    c. Claims made policy

    d. Claims paid policy

    (Objective 5)

19. In which situation would an employer's liability insurance *not* cover you?

    a. When you did not follow the protocol

    b. When you are volunteering outside of work

    c. When you act based on your own professional judgment

    d. When you are negligent

    (Objective 5)

20. What does the ANA consider a basic nursing liability policy?

    a. $100,000 per claim and $500,000 total

    b. $500,000 per claim and $1,000,000 total

    c. $750,000 per claim and $1,500,000 total

    d. $1,000,000 per claim and $10,000,000 total

    (Objective 5)

21. How is fraud defined?

    a. Attempting to hide covert actions

    b. Misunderstanding the truth

    c. Charting incorrectly

    d. Deceiving deliberately for the purpose of personal gain

    (Objective 6)

22. If a nurse in an emergency situation were to give a patient the lifesaving medicine she believed the physician would order if the physician were present to order it, the nurse would be

    a. acting under the Good Samaritan Act.

    b. guilty of violating the Medical Practice Act.

    c. guilty of violating the Narcotics Act.

    d. assuming expected independence and critical decision-making roles.

    (Objective 6)

23. A nurse who alters a chart entry to prevent anyone from knowing about an error has committed which of the following?

    a. Malpractice

    b. Negligence

    c. Fraud

    d. Defamation of character

    (Objective 6)

24. If you speak about a physician's practice in disapproving and disparaging ways that caused patients to avoid the physician's care, you could be sued for what tort?

    a. Libel

    b. Slander

    c. Breach of confidentiality

    d. Breach of duty

    (Objective 6)

25. Which of the following would *not* be adequate grounds for determining that a person could not give consent?

    a. Dementia

    b. Age 10 years

    c. Age 102 years

    d. Unconsciousness

    (Objective 7)

26. The patient who has given informed consent has done which of the following?

    a. Totally accepted the plan of the treatment

    b. Clearly understood the choices being offered

    c. Had an opportunity to discuss alternatives with the family

    d. Got a second opinion before signing papers

    (Objective 7)

27. A patient who enters the hospital must be informed of what?

    a. The right to make advance directives

    b. Living wills

    c. Durable powers of attorney for health care

    d. Powers of attorney

    (Objective 7)

28. If a person wishes to designate someone to make health care decisions, what document is needed?

    a. A living will

    b. A durable power of attorney for health care

    c. A simple power of attorney

    d. Any advance directive

    (Objective 7)

29. What does negligence consist of?

    a. Doing what one should not have done

    b. Not taking action that one should have taken

    c. Breaking the laws relevant to professional practice

    d. Causing injury by failing to act as a reasonably prudent person

    (Objective 8)

30. Failure to act as a reasonably prudent person would have acted in a specific situation is known as which of the following?

    a. Intentional tort

    b. Malpractice

    c. Negligence

    d. Liability

    (Objective 8)

31. The nursing student is expected to perform to which standard?

    a. Reasonably prudent person

    b. Reasonably prudent nursing student

    c. Reasonably prudent nurse

    d. There is no standard for nursing students.

    (Objective  8)

32. For malpractice to be found, what must be present?

    a. Harm to the patient only

    b. A duty by a professional and harm to the patient

    c. A duty by a professional, a breach of duty, and harm to the patient

    d. A duty by a professional, a breach of duty, harm to the patient, and the breach of duty was the cause of the harm

    (Objective 8)

33. In which situation is a lawsuit most likely?

    a. The patient had a fall with superficial injuries and severe fright that the patient blamed on no one ever answering the call light.

    b. The patient suffered a postoperative infection that extended hospitalization and resulted in a large scar.

    c. The patient was ambulating with a nurse, became suddenly faint, fell, and fractured a wrist.

    d. The patient has a long complicated stay after a heart attack and complains he does not like the food.

    (Objective 9)

34. Which of the following contributes most to suits being filed?

    a. Any error no matter how small

    b. Failure to perceive psychological needs

    c. Serious illness

    d. Incomplete documentation

    (Objective 9)

35. You are the nurse who discovers a patient lying on the floor after a fall. What action should you take *first* to minimize the risk of legal action against the facility or any health care provider?

    a. Record everything you see

    b. Assess the patient and provide emergency care

    c. Be sure a second person is present to verify any action that you take

    d. Call for help to move the patient

    (Objective 9)

36. What is one of the most significant things you can do, as a nurse, to prevent malpractice claims against you?

    a. Carry malpractice insurance

    b. Avoid caring for suit-prone patients

    c. Check with a supervisor before initiating any action

    d. Work at improving your own nursing practice

    (Objective 9)

37. In a court of law, what will best support that you provided high-quality nursing care?

    a. Complete documentation

    b. Testimony of other nurses

    c. Your own testimony

    d. Testimony of a physician

    (Objective 10)

38. When are nurses are considered expert witnesses in court?

    a. They have an advanced degree.

    b. They have worked in nursing for more than 10 years.

    c. They are certified.

    d. They have education and practice experience directly related to the problem being considered.

    (Objective 10)

39. What is a legal testimony that is given and recorded outside of the courtroom?

    a. Writ of habeas corpus

    b. Tort

    c. Deposition

    d. Certified testimony

    (Objective 10)

40. If you are called to testify in court in your capacity as a registered nurse, what should you remember?

    a. You should answer only the questions asked.

    b. You need not tell the entire truth.

c. You are protected by the Good Samaritan statutes.

d. You will always be considered an expert witness.

(Objective 10)

# GAMING IN THE CLASSROOM

*Instructions: This game involves selecting teams and a host. The teams compete against one another for points. Each game has several subject categories. After teams are determined, a team is chosen to go first and selects a category. The host then poses the answer and the team provides the correct question for that answer. Each question can be awarded the same number of points or more difficult questions may be given heavier point values. (The instructor might determine which questions are more difficult based on the content emphasized in class.) Points are awarded to the team that is the first to signal and give a correct question. If that team is incorrect, the other team may attempt to provide the correct question and receive the points. The length of time allowed for response can be determined by the class or by the instructor. The team with the most points at the end of the game is declared the winner. Teams may be composed of individual students or groups of students. Teams may determine their answers as a team or may take turns answering as individuals.*

## Categories

A. Understanding Sources of Law

B. Understanding Liability

C. Advance Directives

D. Types of Torts

## Answers and Questions

### Category A

A: Enacted law and regulatory law.

Q: What is statutory law composed of?

A: Regulatory law.

Q: What type of law is determined by administration agencies of government?

A: Administrative law.

Q: What is another name for regulatory law?

A: Enacted law.

Q: What type of law is passed by the legislature?

A: Composed of common usage, custom, and judicial decision.

Q: What is common law?

A: Ruling.

Q: What is a decision on the law by a judge called?

A: Institutional policy or protocol.

Q: What institutional document might be used to demonstrate common law?

## Category B

A: Negligence.

Q: What is the term for failure to act as a reasonably prudent person?

A: Malpractice.

Q: What is negligence by a professional in the performance of duties called?

A: Respondeat superior.

Q: What is the legal term that indicates the employer or supervisor is liable for acts of an employee?

A: Charitable immunity.

Q: What is the doctrine that limits liability of some charitable institutions?

A: Unintentional tort.

Q: What is harm caused by negligence called?

A: Claims brought insurance.

Q: What type of liability insurance provides protection only if it is in force when the suit is filed?

A: Claims occurred insurance.

Q: What type of liability insurance provides protection even if the policy in force at the time of the incident is no longer in force?

## Category C

A: Living will.

Q: What type of document tells people your wishes in case of a terminal illness?

A: Durable power of attorney for health care.

Q: What type of document gives decision-making authority for health care matters to a specific person?

A: Power of attorney.

Q: What type of document gives authority for financial decision-making to a specific person?

A: Patient Self-Determination Act.

Q: What legislation requires health care facilities or agencies to inform patients of their rights to make advance directives?

A: Informed and voluntary.

Q: What are the two criteria for valid consent?

## Category D

A: Fraud

Q: What is deliberate deception for the purpose of personal gain?

A: Defamation of character.

Q: What is false and malicious communication that is detrimental to a person's reputation?

A: Libel.

Q: What is written defamation of character?

A: Slander.

Q: What is verbal defamation of character?

A: Assault.

Q: What is saying or doing something to make a person genuinely afraid that he or she will be touched without consent.

A: Battery.

Q: What is unwanted or unlawful touching of a person?

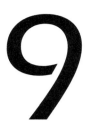

# Ethical Concerns in Nursing Practice

## PURPOSE

This chapter provides a basis for understanding ethical decision making and the concepts pertinent to that process and makes application of those concepts to the health care field. Five ethical theories used when considering ethical problems are presented, and factors that affect ethical decision making are discussed. A framework of ethical decision making is outlined. The chapter concludes with a discussion of ethics applied to patient care and commitment to nursing as a profession, including obligations related to the chemically impaired nursing colleague.

## OBJECTIVES

**1.** Discuss the concept of ethics and its application in the health care field.

**2.** Describe five ethical theories that may be used when considering ethical problems.

**3.** Explain how personal, religious, and philosophical viewpoints, the Code for Nurses, and the Patient's Rights document are used as bases for ethical decision making.

**4.** Discuss how sociocultural and occupational factors affect ethical decision making for nurses.

**5.** Outline a framework for ethical decision making.

**6.** Discuss how ethics relates to commitment to the patient, commitment to personal excellence, and commitment to nursing as a profession.

**7.** Review the ethical and legal obligations related to the chemically impaired nursing colleague.

## KEY TERMS

| | |
|---|---|
| Authoritarian | Morality |
| Autonomy | Mores |
| Beneficence | Natural law |
| Chemical dependency | Nonmaleficence |
| Codes of ethics | Paternalistic |
| Cultural relativism | Social equity |
| Deontology | Teleology |
| Duty | Theory of obligation |
| Ethical dilemma | Utilitarianism |
| Ethics | Values |
| Fidelity | Values clarification |
| Ideal observer theory | Values conflict |
| Justice | Veracity |

## SITUATIONS TO FOSTER CRITICAL THINKING

1. Review the basic ethical concepts presented in your text. Identify at least one clinical situation with which you are familiar where each concept would be applicable. Is more than one concept applicable in each case? Does one take precedence over another? Why? What factors need to be considered? (Objective 1)

2. Compare and contrast the five ethical theories presented in the text. Select the one theory that best accommodates your values. Provide a rationale for selecting that theory as a basis for ethical decision making. Does that theory have any particular weakness? (Objective 2)

3. The Code for Nurses was written in 1973. Review the document. Do you believe it is current for today's practice? Provide the rationale for your response. If you

were going to add or delete content, what would it be? Again provide a rationale for your response. (Objective 3)

4. Give at least four instances in which social and cultural factors affect ethical decision making. How have they affected it? Is it impacted by economic or occupational factors? In what ways are societal values involved? What impact does it have on the population at large? (Objective 4)

5. Denise Martin is employed as charge nurse in a local nursing home. Recently a decision was made to discontinue the tube feedings a comatose patient has been receiving. Some of the staff, particularly the nursing assistants, are very distressed about this order. What can Denise do to assist her staff? Who might help with the problem? How should she begin? What factors will she need to consider? (Objectives 1, 2, 4, and 5)

6. In health care we sometimes do harm to individuals although that is not intended (nonmaleficence). Identify some clinical situations in which this can occur. What will you do as a professional nurse to limit the occurrence of these situations? How will you deal with those that cannot be prevented? (Objectives 1, 5, and 6)

7. Select a particular ethical issue. Identify how you will address that issue and maintain your personal commitment to excellence. (Objective 6)

8. You have been working on the unit for 6 months. Recently you have noticed that a colleague has demonstrated difficulty meeting schedules and deadlines, has done sloppy charting, has had two medication errors of which you are aware, and has had four absences in the last month. Several of the patients also have complained that the pain medication they received did not help their discomfort. What would you think might be the problem? What would you do? Where would you begin? Explain why you chose to take the actions you have outlined. (Objective 7)

## DISCUSSION/ESSAY QUESTIONS

1. Give examples (anonymous) of situations of which you are aware that pose ethical dilemmas in health care. (Objective 1)

2. Explain to a colleague or to your class, the concept of ethics with consideration of its application to health care. (Objective 1)

3. Describe how morals applies to the concept of ethics. (Objective 1)

4. Define the concept of justice from an ethical standpoint. (Objective 2)

5. Describe a situation in which beneficence and autonomy might be in conflict. (Objective 2)

6. Discuss the concept of "rights" and how ensuring that rights of the individual are respected can affect health care delivery. (Objective 2)

7. Select the one basic ethical concept that you believe has the most applicability to the population in general and defend the selection of that concept. (Objective 2)

8. Think of an example from your personal experience in which you believe an individual's (anonymous) right to autonomy was violated. How would you have changed the situation? (Objective 2)

9. Do you believe that beneficence, autonomy, or justice has the strongest claim? Why? (Objective 2)

10. Describe the difference between the concepts of beneficence and nonmaleficence. (Objective 2)

11. Provide an example of the concept of fidelity applied to health care delivery. (Objectives 1 and 2)

12. Discuss what is meant by the "standard of best interest." (Objective 2)

13. Give an example of the application of utilitarianism to health care delivery. Do you believe it was an appropriate application? Why or why not? (Objectives 1 and 2)

14. Give an example of how using Rawl's approach to social justice might affect an ethical decision. (Objective 2)

15. Explain how the decision of an individual using utilitarian ethics would differ from that of an individual taking a position that there are consistent moral truths. (Objective 2)

16. Discuss some of the problems you could anticipate in using the concept of ideal observer as a basis for ethical decision making. (Objective 2)

17. What is the purpose of the American Nurses Association Code for Nurses? (Objective 3)

18. Give at least three examples of how a person's religious beliefs will influence that person's ethical decision making. (Objective 3)

19. Select one item from the Patient's Bill of Rights and describe how one of the bases for ethical decision making applies to that right. (Objectives 1 and 3)

20. Select one item from the International Code for Nurses and describe how one of the bases for ethical decision making applies to that code. (Objectives 1 and 3)

21. Give at least three examples of how a person's social orientation will influence that person's ethical decision making. (Objective 4)

22. How does the law affect ethical decision making? (Objective 4)

23. How have science and technology influenced ethical problems in health care? (Objective 4)

24. How has the paternalistic background of the hospital affected nurses as decision makers in ethical situations? (Objective 4)

25. Identify one situation (anonymous) in which you could apply the framework to ethical decision making outlined in your text. (Objective 5)

26. Of the steps in the framework for ethical decision making is there one step that

you believe is more important than another? If so, why? (Objective 5)

27. Outline a method of self-evaluation that you would feel comfortable using. (Objective 6)

28. Do you believe that nurses should evaluate peers or that evaluation should be performed by supervisors only? Why? (Objective 6)

29. How might you respond to a negative personal evaluation of your nursing performance? (Objective 6)

30. A friend asks you to recommend an obstetrician and you are knowledgeable about the care provided by a number of obstetricians in the area. How would you respond to your friend's request? (Objective 6)

31. What should you do if you believe a colleague in nursing is coming to work under the influence of alcohol? (Objective 7)

32. What resources are available in your community and state to assist a chemically dependent nurse? (Objective 7)

## FILL IN THE BLANKS

*Instructions: Complete the following statements by filling in the blanks with the word or words that make the sentence complete and correct.*

1. In the formal sense, ethics is a branch of philosophy referred to as _____ philosophy. (Objective 1)

2. Societal norms, religion, and family orientation provide the framework for our personal _____. (Objective 1)

3. _____ _____ is a process that includes assessing, exploring, and determining personal values. (Objective 1)

4. The _____ of the individual have been increasingly emphasized in all aspects of living and, more recently, in dying. (Objective 1)

5. The basis of most professional codes and legal judgments is _____. (Objective 1)

6. When we are talking about the right to self-determination, independence, and freedom, we are referring to an individual's _____. (Objective 1)

7. The obligation to do good, not harm, to other people is known as _____. (Objective 1)

8. The prohibition of intentional harm is known as _____. (Objective 1)

9. The obligation to be fair to all people is the concept of _____. (Objective 1)

10. The obligation to be faithful to the agreements, commitments, and responsibilities that one has made to oneself and others is known as _____. (Objective 1)

11. Telling the truth or not intentionally deceiving or misleading patients relates to the concept of _____. (Objective 1)

12. When a decision is based on what the health care providers or family believe is best for that individual, it is done in the _____ __ ____ _____. (Objective 1)

13. When a unilateral decision is made by a health care provider for a patient without input from the patient or family, it may be viewed as _____. (Objective 1)

14. A moral principle or a set of moral principles that can be used in assessing what is morally right or morally wrong is a (an) _____ _____. (Objective 2)

15. The ethical theory that states that an act is right if it is useful in bringing about a desirable or good outcome for the greatest number is _____. (Objective 2)

16. Rawl's approach to justice focuses on the concept of _____ _____. (Objective 2)

17. St. Thomas Aquinas is credited with developing the theory of _____ ____. (Objective 2)

18. Two documents developed by nurses that provide common guidelines to use in making ethical decisions are the _____ ___ _____ and the _____ _____ _____ ___ _____. (Objective 3)

19. A document published by the American Hospital Association that can provide guidelines for ethical decision making is the _____ __ __ _____. (Objective 3)

20. A major avenue for debating and trying to solve ethical problems is provided through our _____ _____. (Objective 4)

21. Of major concern to our society as a whole is the issue of _____ of health care. (Objective 4)

22. Relationships among nurses who work together in which they support one another, share in decision making, and present a unified approach to problems are called _____relationships. (Objective 5)

23. Two factors in the background of hospital governance have contributed to nurses not being decision makers. These two factors are the _____ and _____ backgrounds. (Objective 5)

24. A hospital committee established to assist individuals who must make ethical decisions and to work in an advisory way with medical staff members is the _____ committee. (Objective 4)

25. The first step in the basic framework for ethical decision making involves _____ and _____ the ethical problem. (Objective 5)

26. Most ethical problems have more than one possible _____. (Objective 5)

27. Nursing has a long history of _____ to the well-being of patients who need care. (Objective 6)

28. Making a severely critical remark to a patient about a physician's practice could result in a legal charge of _____. (Objective 6)

29. The first step in any situation in which you believe substandard care exists is to collect adequate and valid _____. (Objective 6)

30. When dealing with substandard care, it is critical that you understand the system of _____ and _____ within your facility. (Objective 6)

31. To meet the commitment to a patient, each individual nurse must be committed to personal _____. (Objective 6)

32. Ensuring that your personal practices are what they should be means that you will be involved in _____. (Objective 6)

33. Stealing a small amount or stealing objects of little value is known as _____. (Objective 6)

34. A planned program of evaluation that includes ongoing monitoring of the care given and of outcomes of care is known as _____ _____. (Objective 6)

35. The first aspect of nursing care that is usually evaluated is whether nursing actions taken are _____ and _____. (Objective 6)

36. Specific, observable patient behaviors or clinical manifestations that are the desired results of care are known as _____ _____. (Objective 6)

37. Quality assurance programs are required of hospitals by the _____ _____ __ __ _____ __ _____ _____. (Objective 6)

38. The term used to describe a person whose practice has deteriorated because of chemical abuse is _____ _____. (Objective 7)

39. Problems related to drug abuse are complicated by the fact that the nurse usually is obtaining drugs _____ _____ _____. (Objective 7)

40. If you suspect that a colleague has a chemical dependency problem, the first thing you need to do is _____ _____ _____ _____ _____ _____ _____ _____. (Objective 7)

# TRUE-FALSE QUESTIONS

*Instructions: Mark the following statements "T" if true or "F" if false. If using a scoring card, mark "A" if true or "B" if false.*

_____ 1. Deciding to participate in providing care for clients who are having abortions is primarily an ethical issue rather than a legal issue. (Objective 1)

_____ 2. Values clarification is a process of assessing, exploring, and determining one's own personal values. (Objective 1)

_____ 3. Morality refers to the rightness or wrongness of an action but is unrelated to society's mores or customs. (Objective 1)

_____ 4. Few guiding principles exist in the health care arena to assist us with ethical decision making. (Objective 1)

_____ 5. Values are most commonly derived from societal norms, religion, and family orientation. (Objective 1)

_____ 6. An ethical dilemma occurs when an individual must make a choice between two equally unfavorable alternatives. (Objective 1)

_____ 7. The "rights" of an individual are seldom extended to include privileges, concessions, and freedoms. (Objective 1)

_____ 8. The Patient Self-Determination Act requires that agencies receiving Medicare money ask patients whether they have advance directives and inform patients of their right to refuse treatment. (Objective 1)

_____ 9. Cultural relativism embraces the notion that groups and individuals hold different sets of values that must be respected. (Objectives 1 and 4)

_____ 10. Autonomy refers to the right of self-determination, independence, and freedom. (Objective 1)

_____ 11. Beneficence refers to the obligation to be fair to all people. (Objective 1)

_____ 12. Nonmaleficence refers to the obligation to be faithful to the agreements, commitments, and responsibilities that one has made to oneself and others. (Objective 1)

_____ 13. Veracity refers to telling the truth or not intentionally deceiving or misleading patients. (Objective 1)

_____ 14. Health care providers strive to avoid unilateral decisions made by a health care provider.

_____ 15. Most ethical theories cannot be adapted to situations that we encounter in the health care delivery system. (Objective 2)

_____ 16. An example of deontology might be applied to a situation in which all persons involved in the research study have a complete understanding of the study and its purposes. (Objective 2)

_____ 17. Few people rely on formal philosophical or religious beliefs that define matters in relation to what is believed to be the truth or good or evil. (Objective 3)

_____ 18. Ethical decisions are most frequently made without consideration of other factors, such as personal, religious, or philosophical viewpoints because these viewpoints tend to cloud the issue. (Objective 3)

_____ 19. The *ANA Code for Nurses* is legally binding. (Objective 3)

_____ 20. The *International Council of Nurses Code for Nurses* is not used by nurses in the United States because there is a national code in the United States. (Objective 3)

_____ 21. The rights outlined in the *American Hospital Association's A Patient's Bill of Rights* identifies penalties for hospitals that fail to ensure patients these rights. (Objective 3)

_____ 22. The *American Hospital Association's Patient's Bill of Rights* is legally binding on all hospitals that are members of that association. (Objective 3)

_____ 23. The size of the group being affected by ethical decision has little to do with the decision-making process. (Objective 4)

_____ 24. The value a society places on the individual or the family directly influences the standard of care. (Objective 4)

_____ 25. A culture's religious values and belief in an afterlife directly affect ethical issues. (Objective 4)

_____ 26. The judicial system has little impact on ethical decision making. (Objective 4)

_____ 27. By formalizing reasons and procedures for termination of employment and outlining grievance measures, a contract may provide nurses greater freedom. (Objective 6)

_____ 28. Today, nurses are seldom represented on hospital ethics committees. (Objective 6)

_____ 29. The paternalistic background of the hospital has supported nurses as decision makers. (Objective 6)

_____ 30. The authoritarian background of the hospital has limited nurses as decision makers. (Objective 6)

_____ 31. Nurses demonstrate commitment to excellence by participating in ethics committees. (Objective 6)

_____ 32. Nurses are seldom in the position of being asked to recommend a physician or other type of care provider. (Objective 6)

_____ 33. A final alternative to a problem in your work setting is to offer your resignation if the change is not made. (Objective 6)

_____ 34. If we work long enough and seriously enough with ethical dilemmas, it is possible to arrive at decisions that will be acceptable to all parties involved. (Objective 6)

_____ 35. Most ethical problems have more than one possible solution. (Objectives 5 and 6)

_____ 36. The day has passed when nurses could be expected to provide unwavering support of all members of the health care team. (Objective 7)

_____ 37. In situations in which poor care is being investigated, professional confidentiality may make it seem that nothing is being done. (Objective 7)

_____ 38. In reporting poor care it is critical that your perceptions are correct and that you are well-grounded in your concerns. (Objective 7)

_____ 39. The nursing process format is an inappropriate approach to self-evaluation. (Objective 7)

_____ 40. All hospitals expect that employees will take home bandages and other small items and budget for that. (Objective 7)

## MATCHING QUESTIONS

_Instructions: Match the numbered items with the most appropriate lettered items._

## Group A (Objective 1)

_____ 1. Justice

_____ 2. Veracity

_____ 3. Beneficence

_____ 4. Autonomy

_____ 5. Fidelity

_____ 6. Nonmaleficence

a. The obligation to do good, not harm, to people.

b. The right to make one's own decisions.

c. The prohibition of intentional harm.

d. The obligation to be fair to all people.

e. The obligation to be faithful to the agreements and responsibilities that one has undertaken.

e. Telling the truth.

## Group B (Objective 2)

_____ 1. Social equity and justice

_____ 2. Utilitarianism

_____ 3. Natural law

_____ 4. Deontology

_____ 5. Ideal observer

a. An act is right if it is useful in bringing about a good outcome or end.

b. An ethical theory based on a concept of moral duty or obligation.

c. Actions are morally right when they are in accord with our nature and end as human beings.

d. Requires that decisions be made from a disinterested, dispassionate point of view.

e. An approach to ethics that supports the person most disadvantaged by the situation.

## Group C (Objectives 1, 3, and 4)

_____ 1. Something that is owed to an individual.

_____ 2. A type of ethics that focuses on what people actually do in given situations.

_____ 3. Custom or habit.

_____ 4. Derived from societal norms, religion, and family orientation.

_____ 5. A process that fosters the identification of factors we believe are important.

_____ 6. Having to make a choice between two equally unfavorable alternatives.

   a. Mores

   b. Values clarification

   c. Descriptive ethics

   d. Ethical dilemma

   e. Values

   f. Rights

## Group D (Objective 2)

_____ 1. Requires that individuals be treated equally regardless of race, sex, marital status, medical diagnosis, social standing, economic level, or religious belief.

_____ 2. All rights and judgments must be able to be applied to all cultures.

_____ 3. Decisions based on the individual's expressed wishes or on documents such as living wills.

_____ 4. A moral principle or a set of moral principles that can be used to assess what is morally right or wrong in a given situation.

_____ 5. The concept that good should be promoted and evil avoided.

_____ 6. When we must choose between two things, both of which are important to us.

   a. Natural law

   b. Values conflict

   c. Ethical theory

   d. Distributive justice

   e. Standard of best interest

   f. Cultural relativism

## MULTIPLE-CHOICE QUESTIONS

_Instructions: Choose the one best answer for each question._

1. The discipline of ethics can be divided into three areas comprised of meta-ethics, normative ethics, and which of the following?

   a. Descriptive ethics

   b. Focused ethics

   c. Humanistic ethics

   d. Rational ethics

   (Objective 1)

2. Which of the following is characteristic of values?

   a. They are fairly uniform throughout the world.

   b. Each of us has a differing set of values.

   c. By and large, our values remain unchanged throughout our lifetime.

   d. Religion and philosophy have little impact on values.

   (Objective 1)

3. Which of the following best defines the term _mores_?

   a. Behavior that is good, right, honorable, or desirable.

   b. Behavior that is bad, wrong, improper, or irresponsible.

c. Custom or habit.

d. Learned habits.

(Objective 1)

4. Which of the following is a reason we do values clarification?

   a. It is a required part of most social science curricula.

   b. It is expected in today's society.

   c. It is a mandatory part of all nursing curricula.

   d. It assists us to have a better understanding of ourselves.

   (Objective 1)

5. Which of the following represents the obligation to be faithful to the agreements and responsibilities one has undertaken?

   a. Beneficence

   b. Fidelity

   c. Justice

   d. Veracity

   (Objective 1)

6. A nurse believes that the primary consideration in working with a group of patients is that any decision must be fair to all. Which concept of ethics does this attitude represent?

   a. Autonomy

   b. Beneficence

   c. Justice

   d. Utility

   (Objective 1)

7. A nurse believes that it is very important to let patients make their own decisions. Which ethical concept does this attitude represent?

   a. Autonomy

   b. Beneficence

   c. Justice

d. Utility

(Objective 1)

8. A nurse believes that the most important consideration is that no harm be done to the patient. Which ethical concept does this attitude represent?

   a. Autonomy

   b. Beneficence

   c. Justice

   d. Utility

   (Objective 1)

9. Which of the following ethical concepts provides the foundation for the nurse's accountability?

   a. Beneficence

   b. Fidelity

   c. Justice

   d. Utility

   (Objective 1)

10. When honest and straightforward answers are not provided to a patient, which of the following ethical concepts is being violated?

    a. Beneficence

    b. Fidelity

    c. Justice

    d. Veracity

    (Objective 1)

11. Which ethical theory supports the concept that an act is right if it brings about the greatest good for the greatest number?

    a. Deontology

    b. Natural law

    c. Social equity and justice

    d. Utilitarianism

    (Objective 2)

12. Which of the following best describes Rawl's position on ethics?

    a. An act is good if it brings the greatest good to the greatest number.

    b. Decisions are based on unchanging principles and moral rules.

    c. Actions are right when they are in accord with our nature.

    d. A reasonable person would support the alternative that favored the most disadvantaged person.

    (Objective 2)

13. A decision to use available funds to help the greatest number, regardless of seriousness of illness or need, would be most consistent with which philosophical position?

    a. Utilitarianism

    b. Categorical imperative of Kant

    c. Social justice

    d. Making a decision from a dispassionate point of view

    (Objective 3)

14. Which of the following statements is true of ethical concerns in nursing?

    a. Nurses are not expected to make ethical decisions.

    b. Correct ethical decisions are outlined in the *ANA Code for Nurses*.

    c. Increasing technology has resulted in situations for which there are no clear-cut answers.

    d. Nurses are participants in all ethical decisions that affect their practice.

    (Objectives 3 and 4)

15. What a patient can expect in care is often found in documents identifying the patient's rights. Which of the following is one such document?

    a. Accreditation standards

    b. Codes of ethics

    c. Position papers

    d. Utilization reviews

    (Objectives 1 and 3)

16. Which of the following is one method used to help assess, explore, and determine our personal values?

    a. Meditation

    b. Mediation

    c. Consciousness raising

    d. Values clarification

    (Objective 1)

17. Which of the following provides guidelines accepted by the nursing profession as a whole for use in making ethical decisions?

    a. Hippocratic Oath

    b. Morse code

    c. *ANA Code for Nurses*

    d. *Encyclopedia of Bioethics*

    (Objective 3)

18. Who authored the *Patient's Bill of Rights*?

    a. American Medical Association

    b. American Hospital Association

    c. American Nurses Association

    d. Department of Health and Human Services

    (Objective 3)

19. Which group developed the *Code for Nurses*?

    a. National League for Nursing

    b. National Student Nurses Association

    c. American Medical Association

    d. American Nurses Association

    (Objective 3)

20. Which of the following groups of individuals is demanding greater involvement in all aspects of health care?

    a. Consumers

    b. Hospital medical staffs

    c. Nurse practitioners

    d. Third-party payers

    (Objectives 3 and 4)

21. What is the major effect that increasing scientific knowledge and technology in health care have had on ethical decision making?

    a. Decisions may now be made by computers, which are impartial.

    b. Greater technology allows us to put off decisions about death because it can be forestalled.

    c. More complex procedures have all been accompanied by complex ethical concerns.

    d. No basic changes in the ethical questions in health care have been caused by technology.

    (Objective 4)

22. Historically, why have nurses, most of whom are women, been relegated to dependent and subservient roles?

    a. Collective bargaining contracts

    b. Their unwillingness to be involved

    c. The lack of men in nursing

    d. The authoritarian and paternalistic attitudes of physicians and hospitals

    (Objective 4)

23. Which of the following most affects the ability of nurses to be autonomous decision makers regarding ethical questions?

    a. Status of the employee

    b. Lack of specific courses in ethics in the basic program

    c. Limited involvement in situations that require ethical decisions

    d. The collegial support of other nurses

    (Objectives 4 and 6)

24. Which of the following factors impinges on the nurse's autonomy in ethical decision making?

    a. Authoritarian and paternalistic background of hospitals

    b. Limitations imposed in licensure requirements

    c. Guidelines specified in collective bargaining agreements

    d. Lack of knowledge about ethics

    (Objectives 4 and 6)

25. When identifying or clarifying an ethical problem, which of the following will you want to determine first?

    a. What decision must be made

    b. Who will make the decision

    c. When you must make the decision

    d. Why you need to make a decision

    (Objective 5)

26. Which of the following is true of ethical dilemmas?

    a. In most instances there is an obvious answer.

    b. In most instances there is only one answer.

    c. It is impossible to know what will be the best answer.

    d. In most instances problems have more than one possible answer.

    (Objective 5)

27. Which of the following is true in many ethical situations?

    a. Outcomes are predictable.

    b. Unforeseen outcomes are common.

c. Outcomes from one situation are not applicable to another.

d. Outcomes cannot be assessed while you are proceeding.

(Objective 5)

28. Which of the following is a reason nurses are frequently asked to recommend a care provider?

   a. The public knows they will always get good advice.

   b. The public knows you will give them the "straight scoop."

   c. The public doesn't know where else to ask.

   d. The public believes that you have special knowledge and insight into such matters.

   (Objective 6)

29. Which response to a request for information regarding a care provider would be ethically and legally appropriate?

   a. Dr. James is a honey—and cute, too.

   b. Dr. Madison is a terror. I wouldn't let him take care of my dog, much less my child.

   c. Dr. Johnson usually encourages parent participation in care while a child is hospitalized.

   d. No doctor is as good as Dr. Wilson.

   (Objective 6)

30. Which is the first step you should take if you believe substandard care exists?

   a. Confront the caregiver personally.

   b. Discuss your concerns with your immediate supervisor.

   c. Tell the client you believe she or he has been the recipient of poor care.

   d. Collect adequate, valid information.

   (Objective 6)

31. Which of the following is an essential step in achieving personal excellence in practice?

   a. Thorough and conscientious self-evaluation

   b. Continuing your education toward a higher degree

   c. Serving as a mentor for a newer graduate

   d. Serving on a hospital policy committee

   (Objective 6)

32. If you observe an error in nursing care given by a peer, which of the following is an appropriate first action?

   a. Submit a written report to your immediate supervisor.

   b. Speak with the nurse privately about your concern.

   c. Correct the mistake, but say nothing.

   d. Ignore the situation; each nurse is responsible for her or his own practice.

   (Objective 6)

33. What is the first step in self-evaluation?

   a. Gathering data

   b. Identifying problems

   c. Asking for feedback from others

   d. Setting up a plan for continuing education

   (Objective 6)

34. What is the term by which we refer to a method of evaluating nursing care by examination of records only?

   a. Accreditation

   b. Audit

   c. Quality assurance

   d. Peer review

   (Objective 6)

35. By what term do we refer to criteria that describe the result of care as seen in the patient?

    a. Detail criteria

    b. Evaluation criteria

    c. Outcome criteria

    d. Process criteria

    (Objective 6)

36. What is the term used to refer to criteria that describe the correct and complete actions to be taken by health care providers?

    a. Detail criteria

    b. Evaluation criteria

    c. Outcome criteria

    d. Process criteria

    (Objective 6)

37. What is the first step you should take if you suspect that a nursing peer is practicing under the influence of alcohol?

    a. Confront the individual personally.

    b. Talk with your immediate supervisor in an informal way.

    c. Ask to transfer to another unit to avoid legal liability.

    d. Record specific dates and behaviors observed.

    (Objective 7)

38. You are working days and have noted that whenever a certain nurse works nights, the postoperative patients complain of unrelieved pain and very restless nights. What would be the first thing you should do?

    a. Tell the nurse involved what you have observed and that you will be watching the situation closely.

    b. Suggest to the head nurse that the nurse in question be transferred to the day shift where more nurses are around to observe her behavior.

    c. Document specific dates, patients, drugs given, and patient responses.

    d. Tell the head nurse that nurse X is using drugs and should be dismissed.

    (Objective 7)

39. In addition to concerns that the chemically impaired nurse may injure patients, what might be another concern?

    a. The liability of working with someone who is chemically impaired

    b. Personal concern for the nurse who is afflicted

    c. The staffing during the time the nurse is left off the unit

    d. That the Board of Nursing might learn of the problem

    (Objective 7)

## GAMING IN THE CLASSROOM

*Instructions: This game involves selecting teams and a host. The teams compete against one another for points. Each game has several subject categories. After teams are determined, a team is chosen to go first and selects a category. The host then poses the answer and the team provides the correct question for that answer. Each question can be awarded the same number of points or more difficult questions may be given heavier point values. (The instructor might determine which questions are more difficult based on the content emphasized in class.) Points are awarded to the team that is the first to signal and give a correct question. If that team is incorrect, the other team may attempt to provide the correct question and receive the points. The length of time allowed for response can be determined by the class or by the instructor. The team with the most points at the end of the game is declared the winner. Teams may be composed of individual students or groups of students. Teams may determine their answers as a team or may take turns answering as individuals.*

## Categories

A. Ethical Concepts

B. Ethical Theories

C. Codes and Rights

D. Factors Influencing Decision Making

E. Professional Practice

## Answers and Questions

### Category A

A: Something we think of as an entitlement or as owed to the individual.

Q: What are rights?

A: Involves the right of self-determination, independence, and freedom.

Q: What is autonomy?

A: Refers to the obligation to be fair to all people.

Q: What is justice?

A: Refers to the obligation to be faithful to the agreements, commitments, and responsibilities one has made to oneself and to others.

Q: What is fidelity?

A: Refers to telling the truth and no intentional deceiving or misleading patients.

Q: What is veracity?

### Category B

A: An act is right when it brings the greatest good to the greatest number.

Q: What is utilitarianism?

A: Ethical decision making is based on moral rules and unchanging principles for motivations that are derived from universal values.

Q: What is deontology?

A: Actions are morally right when they are in accord with our nature and end as human beings.

Q: What is natural law?

A: If people of reason were placed in a situation of ethical choice, they would choose the alternative that supported the most disadvantaged person.

Q: What is the theory of social equity and justice?

A: Requires that decisions be made from a disinterested, dispassionate, omniscient viewpoint.

Q: What is the theory of the ideal observer?

### Category C

A: Has been referred to as "the most interesting and responsive code I have ever read" by the editor-in-chief of the *Encyclopedia of Bioethics*.

Q: What is the Code for Nurses?

A: Was written in 1973 and revised in 1989.

Q: What is the International Council of Nurses Code?

A: Was published by the American Hospital Association.

Q: What is a Patient's Bill of Rights?

A: An act that established the right of citizens to know that certain information is available in a record system.

Q: What is the Federal Privacy Act?

A: A report published by the Institute of Medicine in 1995 recommending assurance of confidentiality and protection of privacy rights.

Q: What is Health Data in the Information Age?

### Category D

A: The size of the group being affected by ethical decisions has a bearing on the decision-making process.

Q: What is a social factor affecting decision making?

A: Belief in an afterlife is an example.

Q: What is a religious value that affects individual decision making?

A: The development of the kidney dialysis machine is an example.

Q: What is scientific advancement and technology?

A: A greater acceptance of infants born to single mothers was instrumental in bringing this about.

Q: What is legislation that changed the wording on birth certificates to drop the word *illegitimate*?

A: Issues are taken to court where they are debated.

Q: What results in judicial decision making?

## Category E

A: A term that refers to stealing in small amounts or stealing objects of little value.

Q: What is pilfering?

A: The first step you should take if you are in a situation in which you believe substandard care exists.

Q: What is collect adequate, valid information and be sure of your facts?

A: Is a planned program of evaluation that included ongoing monitoring of the care given and of outcomes of care.

Q: What is quality assurance?

A: Could serve as one approach to the self-evaluation.

Q: What is the nursing process format?

A: Is a term used to describe that person whose practice has deteriorated because of chemical abuse.

Q: What is the chemically impaired professional?

# 10

# Bioethical Issues in Health Care

## PURPOSE

This chapter exposes the student to some of the many bioethical issues emerging in health care today. Included are topics such as family planning practices, abortion, in vitro fertilization, genetic screening, and surrogate motherhood. The chapter also covers issues related to dying, such as active euthanasia and passive euthanasia, the problems related to securing organs for donations, xenotransplantation, and informed consent and treatment. The chapter concludes with a discussion of the treatment of the mentally ill.

## OBJECTIVES

1. Discuss major bioethical issues and give examples of nursing involvement.

2. Outline the history of family planning practices in the United States and discuss how various value systems and beliefs have affected it.

3. Analyze the controversy surrounding the Human Genome Project and its relationship to genetic screening.

4. List some of the possible ethical and legal problems associated with artificial insemination, surrogate motherhood, and in vitro fertilization.

5. Discuss the problems associated with determining when death has occurred.

6. Review and examine multiple factors in right-to-die issues, including the difference between active euthanasia and passive euthanasia.

7. Discuss the major issues related to withholding or withdrawing treatment, and patients' rights with regard to informed consent and treatment.

8. Identify the major concerns associated with organ transplantation.

9. Discuss the factors that make it difficult to establish firm rules regarding the treatment of the mentally ill.

10. Outline concerns related to the rationing of health care.

## KEY TERMS

Abortion (spontaneous, therapeutic, elective)
Advance directives
Age of consent
Amniocentesis
Artificial insemination
Assisted death
Behavior control
Bioethics
Death
Durable power of attorney for health care
Emancipation of a minor
Eugenics
Euthanasia
Genetic mother
Genetics
Genetic screening
Gestational mother
Family planning

Futile treatment
Informed consent
In vitro fertilization
Living will
Mature minor
Negative euthanasia
Negative right simpliciter
Organ procurement
Organ transplantation
Patient self-determination (PSD)
Positive euthanasia
Property rights
Right to die
Spare-the-mother syndrome
Surrogate mother
Withdrawing/ withholding treatment
Wrongful birth
Xenografts/xeno- transplantation

## SITUATIONS TO FOSTER CRITICAL THINKING

1. Think of a situation in which you have been involved as a nursing student when bioethics was a consideration. What information was needed to deal with the situation? Where could that information have been obtained? What was your personal position regarding the issue? How did you reach that position? Was it supported by others? (Objective 1)

2. You are working the night shift on the obstetrics unit. As you make rounds at 1:30 A.M., you find Mrs. Rodder, a Roman Catholic patient who has just delivered her seventh child, crying. As you talk with her, you learn that she does not want to go home the next morning because she is afraid she will be pregnant again within the next year. Giving full consideration to her religious views, what will be your response to her concern? (Objective 2)

3. What social and legal concerns can you identify with regard to the Human Genome Project? What might be the worst situation that could evolve? What might be the best? How might these concerns be mitigated? (Objective 3)

4. If you were given the assignment of developing guidelines for the practice of using a surrogate mother, what criteria would you establish? How would you ensure that these criteria were carried out? To whom would you assign this responsibility? (Objective 4)

5. Your sister and her husband have been unable to conceive a child although they have been trying for 7 years. She asks you about the pros and cons of in vitro fertilization and what it involves. What would you tell her? Discuss this with a classmate and determine whether the classmate would add or subtract anything from what you would share. Why? (Objective 4)

6. What issues have resulted in difficulty determining when death has occurred? If you were serving on a hospital ethics committee, what recommendations would you make that would help eliminate or mitigate some of these problems? (Objective 5)

7. Mr. Allen is preparing for discharge following recovery from a serious heart attack. He and his wife are interested in learning more about durable power of attorney in the event that the family has serious problems in the future. What information would you provide to them? To whom would you refer the family? What would be the major considerations? (Objective 6)

8. Examine the various position papers on withholding or withdrawing treatment. Which one do you believe gives the best direction or assistance? Why? What recommendations would you have regarding strengthening the other positions? (Objective 7)

9. As a nurse on the pediatric unit, you are helping to admit 11-year-old Bryan who is scheduled for surgery to have a benign, but very unattractive growth removed from his right thigh. His parents have signed the surgery permit. While talking with Bryan he tells you he really does not want to have the surgery. Further conversation with him supports his seriousness with regard to this matter. How would you proceed? (Objective 7)

10. You have been selected to serve on a committee that must make a decision with regard to which one of three patients who are awaiting a heart transplant will get the organ that has just become available. All three patients are critical and may not live until another organ becomes available. What criteria would you use for making your decision? (Objective 8)

11. What benefits do you see with xenographs? What disadvantages exist? Do the benefits outweigh the disadvantages? Why or why not? (Objective 8)

12. Do you believe the federal government should invest large amounts of money in research related to the development of artificial organs, such as kidneys, hearts, or livers? Give the reasons for your response. If it is yes, how would you propose that this be funded? (Objective 8)

13. The guidelines for treatment of the mentally ill are now 17 years old. Do you believe they are still current? If not, how would you suggest they be changed? (Objective 9)

14. What do you see as the greatest problems associated with the rationing of health care? Are these serious enough that health care should not be rationed? What solutions could you propose? (Objective 10)

## DISCUSSION/ESSAY QUESTIONS

1. Discuss what is meant by the word *bioethics*. (Objective 1)

2. Which bioethical issues cause us the most concern and why? (Objective 1)

3. Why have bioethical concerns increased in the last 10 years? (Objective 1)

4. Discuss the position of the Roman Catholic Church on birth control. (Objective 2)

5. How does the age of consent affect decision making with regard to bioethical issues? (Objective 2)

6. Cite at least two reasons why a family may not wish to practice birth control. (Objective 2)

7. Discuss the arguments in favor of the availability of abortion. (Objective 2)

8. Discuss the arguments against the availability of abortion. (Objective 2)

9. Are there any extenuating circumstances that one who is basically against abortion might consider? If so, what are they? (Objective 2)

10. What is artificial insemination and what are the different ways in which it can be carried out? (Objective 2)

11. What is the major reason for performing an amniocentesis? Do you think there are other reasons that are equally important? (Objective 3)

12. What are the advantages and disadvantages of being able to do an amniocentesis? (Objective 3)

13. Identify some of the conditions that can be diagnosed prenatally via amniocentesis. (Objective 3)

14. Define the term *eugenics* and explain when it was first discussed. (Objective 2)

15. Explain how events that occurred during Hitler's regime resulted in eugenics becoming very unpopular. (Objective 3)

16. Give some arguments supporting the use of in vitro fertilization and some arguments against the use of it. (Objective 3)

17. Cite two concerns that arise when a surrogate mother has been employed to give birth to a baby. (Objective 4)

18. Do you believe that records should be kept on all donor sperm so that a child conceived from artificial insemination using that donor sperm can have access to a genetic history? Defend your position. (Objective 4)

19. Do think becoming a first-time mother after the age of 60 is desirable or undesirable? Give your rationale. (Objective 4)

20. Of the various types of assisted reproductive techniques available, do you believe some are more ethical than others? If so, which ones and why? (Objective 4)

21. Describe death as defined in *Black's Law Dictionary*. (Objective 5)

22. Why is the *Black's Law Dictionary* definition of death no longer adequate to meet the demands of society? (Objective 5)

23. What is currently accepted as a definition of death? (Objective 5)

24. Identify some situations in which persons might support negative euthanasia. (Objective 6)

25. Differentiate between positive euthanasia and negative euthanasia. (Objective 6)

26. What is the purpose of the living will? (Objective 7)

27. Do you believe laws should be passed requiring that all persons have implemented the paperwork necessary for power of attorney for health care? Defend your position. (Objective 7)

28. What are the rights of the patient with regard to informed consent? (Objective 7)

29. Identify at least one situation in which it would be appropriate to withhold treatment. (Objective 7)

30. How does the concept of withholding treatment differ from that of withdrawing treatment? (Objective 7)

31. Are there any circumstances under which you believe it is appropriate to withdraw nourishment? Explain your answer. (Objective 7)

32. Provide a definition of behavior control as it is used in the treatment of the mentally ill. (Objective 9)

33. Why is anything that smacks of behavior control regarded with suspicion in our society? (Objective 9)

34. What are some of the major guidelines that have been proposed for dealing with the area of behavior control? (Objective 9)

35. What is electroconvulsive therapy and why are some persons opposed to it? (Objective 9)

36. Identify some of the objections to the control of behavior through pharmacologic agents. (Objective 9)

37. Identify some of the objections to the control of behavior through psychotherapy. (Objective 9)

38. How is society dealing with the problem of scarce medical resources? (Objective 10)

39. Outline the concerns related to rationing of care. (Objective 10)

40. If you were responsible for determining who would receive care and to what degree, what criteria would you use for making your decisions? (Objective 10)

## FILL IN THE BLANKS

*Instructions: Complete the following statements by filling in the blanks with the word or words that make the sentence complete and correct.*

1. _____ is the study of ethical issues that result from technological and scientific advances. (Objective 1)

2. The Institute of Society, Ethics, and the Life Sciences, located in Hastings-on-Hudson, is an example of a _____ __ _____ in bioethics. (Objective 1)

3. Many bioethical issues are the product of the _____ _____ that have occurred in medical practice and research. (Objective 1)

4. Hearts from genetically altered pigs were transplanted into baboons in _____, proving that cross-species transplantations can be done. (Objectives 1 and 8).

5. In 1893, Congress passed the Comstock Act prohibiting the sale, mailing, or importation of any drug or article that _____ _____. (Objective 2)

6. A clear legal concept of planned parenthood was not developed until _____ when the Supreme Court established the right of the individual to obtain medical advice about contraception. (Objective 2)

7. The age at which one is capable of giving deliberate and voluntary agreement is known as the _____ ___ _____. (Objective 2)

8. A youth who is sufficiently mature and intelligent to understand the nature and consequences of a treatment that is for

her or his benefit is termed a (an) _____ _____. (Objective 2)

9. A model act which addresses the issue of consent of minors for health care was developed in 1973 by the _____ _____ __ _____. (Objective 2)

10. When a pregnancy is deliberately interrupted for medical reasons, the abortion is referred to as a (an) _____ abortion. (Objective 2)

11. When a pregnancy is interrupted for personal reasons, it is termed a (an) _____ abortion. (Objective 2)

12. The court case that resulted in the legalization of abortion is known as the _____ ____ _____ decision. (Objective 2)

13. A technique in which approximately 20 mL of fluid is withdrawn from the amniotic sac in the uterus of a pregnant woman is called _____. (Objectives 2 and 3)

14. Cases that result when parents bring suit because a child is born who will not have the same quality of life as other children are known as _____ _____ cases. (Objective 2)

15. The movement devoted to improving the human species through the control of hereditary factors in mating is known as _____. (Objective 3)

16. The movement that encourages increasing the desirable traits in the population by urging "worthy" parents to have more children is known as _____ _____. (Objective 3)

17. A _____ may be defined as all the genetic material in the chromosomes of a particular organism. (Objective 3)

18. The practice by which a woman agrees to bear a child conceived through artificial insemination and to relinquish the baby at birth to others for rearing is known as _____ _____. (Objective 4)

19. The first successful in vitro fertilization occurred in England in _____. (Objective 4)

20. When the husband's sperm is used for artificial insemination of his wife, it is known as _____ insemination. (Objective 4)

21. Until recently, the most widely accepted definition of death was from _____ _____ _____. (Objective 5)

22. Treatments that cannot, within a reasonable possibility, cure, ameliorate, improve, or restore a quality of life that would be satisfactory to the patient are referred to as _____. (Objective 6)

23. The federal act that requires that all Medicare and Medicaid providers inform patients, on admission, of their right to refuse treatment is known as the _____ _____ ____. (Objective 6)

24. One document widely used as an advance directive is the _____ ____. (Objective 6)

25. Literally translated, the term *euthanasia* means _____ _____. (Objective 6)

26. A situation in which no extraordinary or heroic measures are undertaken to sustain life is known as _____ or _____ euthanasia. (Objective 6)

27. A situation in which the physician prescribes, supplies, or administers an agent that results in death is known as _____ or _____ euthanasia. (Objective 6)

28. Withholding treatment could be considered _____ euthanasia. (Objective 6)

29. Key to all guidelines on withholding and withdrawing treatment is whether the patient is legally _____ or _____. (Objective 6)

30. The American Nurses Association states that the nurse should not participate in assisted suicide and views it as a violation of the _____ ___ _____. (Objective 7)

31. When the refusal of medical intervention means that the individual is no longer a patient, it is known as a _____ _____ _____ by bioethicists. (Objective 7)

32. A major issue related to organ transplantation is that of _____. (Objective 8)

33. The situation in which there is an inadequate supply of organs to meet societal needs is referred to as _____ _____ _____. (Objective 8)

34. The fact that organ donations from minorities lags behind those from the white population may be due in part to _____ __ _____ and _____. (Objective 8)

35. The practice of using animal organs, cells, and tissues for transplantation into human beings is known as _____. (Objective 8)

36. Some of the problem related to behavior control centers around the fact that people define _____ _____ in different and sometimes conflicting ways. (Objective 9)

37. One of the most common methods of changing behavior in which nurses are involved is the administration of _____ _____. (Objective 9)

38. A therapy long used to treat severe depression is known as _____ _____. (Objective 9)

39. One of the issues that will receive tremendous attention in the 21st century is the _____ of health care. (Objective 10)

40. One of the reasons we will be dealing with the issue of rationing of health care is because of the _____ of care. (Objective 10)

## TRUE-FALSE QUESTIONS

*Instructions: Mark the following statements "T" if true or "F" if false. If using a scoring card, mark "A" if true or "B" if false.*

_____ 1. *Bioethics* is sometimes also called *biomedical ethics*. (Objective 1)

_____ 2. Bioethical issues surrounding the delivery of health care are always clear and straightforward. (Objective 1)

_____ 3. One of the reasons we are confronted with bioethical issues is because our population is getting older and living longer. (Objective 1)

_____ 4. Many of the bioethical issues with which we wrestle have been concerns for many years. (Objective 1)

_____ 5. The Catholic Church believes strongly that the natural use of reproductive powers ensures the propagation of the race. (Objective 2)

_____ 6. The age at which one may consent to treatment and the age at which one can refuse treatment are the same. (Objective 2)

_____ 7. The legal aspects of abortion were not clarified until January 1983. (Objective 2)

_____ 8. There will be times when physicians' ethical and moral convictions prevent them from complying with certain aspects of care. (Objective 2)

_____ 9. Abortion is the termination of pregnancy before viability of the fetus. (Objective 2)

_____ 10. No one objects to abortion when it terminates a pregnancy that results from rape or incest. (Objective 2)

_____ 11. With increasing frequency, voluntary sterilizations have been requested by couples for purposes of terminating reproductive ability. (Objective 2)

_____ 12. Artificial insemination is a newly introduced procedure. (Objective 2)

_____ 13. One major disadvantage of amniocentesis is that it cannot be done until the 36th week of gestation. (Objectives 2 and 3)

_____ 14. Eugenics is a concept that is at least as old as Plato. (Objective 3)

_____ 15. The Human Genome Project was inspired by the discovery that an estimated 4,000 disease genes reside with the human genome. (Objective 3)

_____ 16. The Human Genome Project makes no promises regarding improved diagnosis and treatment of many inherited diseases. (Objective 3)

_____ 17. Few couples view in vitro fertilization as a viable option if they are unable to conceive under normal circumstances. (Objective 3)

_____ 18. Minors of any age can give consent for diagnosis and care of sexually transmitted disease. (Objectives 2 and 7)

_____ 19. Ethicists have little concern that the government might make diagnostic amniocentesis and abortion of all defective fetuses mandatory. (Objectives 2 and 3)

_____ 20. Most states have laws forbidding voluntary sterilization for contraceptive purposes. (Objective 2)

_____ 21. The idea of improving the quality of the human race is at least as old as Plato. (Objective 3)

_____ 22. Eugenics is the movement devoted to improving the human species through genetic control. (Objective 3)

_____ 23. Today there are no states that still allow compulsory eugenic sterilization. (Objectives 3 and 4)

_____ 24. Newer definitions of death have been built around the concept of human potential. (Objective 5)

_____ 25. It is a generally accepted fact that all parts of the body die simultaneously. (Objective 5)

_____ 26. The determination of whether treatment is futile is not difficult now that new standards have been developed. (Objective 6)

_____ 27. In an attempt to gain greater control over the area of dying, many people are now completing a variety of documents that have been titled advance directives. (Objective 7)

_____ 28. The living will and durable power of attorney for health care are essentially the same thing. (Objective 7)

_____ 29. The American Nurses Association supports the concept of assisted suicide because it is a humane way to deal with intractable pain. (Objective 7)

_____ 30. Negative euthanasia refers to a situation in which the physician prescribes, supplies, or administers an agent that results in death. (Objective 6)

_____ 31. There have been no statements or positions issued with regard to withdrawing or withholding treatment. (Objective 7)

_____ 32. Withholding treatment could be considered negative euthanasia. (Objectives 6 and 7)

_____ 33. Nurses who have worked to preserve the patient's dignity have great difficulty "letting go" if a decision is made to withdraw treatment. (Objective 7)

_____ 34. The right to refuse treatment is an issue closely aligned with the right to die. (Objective 7)

_____ 35. The steps to be taken when an individual remains in a persistent vegetative state are clear and straightforward. (Objective 7)

_____ 36. Physicians are in agreement about how much patients should know about their condition. (Objective 7)

_____ 37. In many ways, the ability to use organs for transplantation has required a clearer definition of death. (Objective 8)

_____ 38. The patient is the only one who can give permission for the removal of organs at the time of death. (Objective 8)

_____ 39. We can now change behavior by a variety of methods. (Objective 9)

_____ 40. In many states citizens are being asked to make informed decisions about the rationing of health care. (Objective 10)

## MATCHING QUESTIONS

*Instructions: Match the numbered items with the most appropriate lettered items.*

### Group A (Objectives 2 and 7)

_____ 1. Emancipation of a minor

_____ 2. Informed consent

_____ 3. Paternalism

_____ 4. Age of consent

_____ 5. Mature minor

    a. The age at which one is capable of giving deliberate and voluntary agreement.

    b. A youth who is sufficiently mature and intelligent to understand the nature and consequences of a treatment.

    c. A child legally under the age of majority who is recognized as having the legal capacity of an adult under circumstances prescribed by state law.

    d. The right to know what treatment will be administered.

    e. The locus of decision making is moved from the patient to the physician.

### Group B (Objectives 3 and 6)

_____ 1. Negative euthanasia

_____ 2. Positive euthanasia

_____ 3. Negative eugenics

_____ 4. Positive eugenics

    a. The elimination of unwanted characteristics from a population by discouraging "unworthy" parents.

    b. The increase of desirable traits in a population by urging "worthy" parents to have children.

    c. A situation in which medication is administered to hasten death.

    d. A situation in which no heroic measures are taken to prevent death.

### Group C (Objectives 2, 3, 7, and 8)

_____ 1. Eugenics

_____ 2. Genome

_____ 3. Age of consent

_____ 4. Xenographs

_____ 5. Gene therapy

_____ 6. Competent

    a. All the genetic material in the chromosomes of a particular organism.

    b. Animal-organ transplants.

    c. Able to make decisions for self.

    d. The movement devoted to improving the human species through genetic control.

    e. The age at which one is capable of giving deliberate and voluntary agreement.

    f. The identification and isolation of defective genes, and the replacement with functional genes.

## Group D (Objectives 3 and 4)

_____ 1. Amniocentesis

_____ 2. Prenatal diagnosis

_____ 3. In vitro fertilization

_____ 4. Genetic screening

_____ 5. Artificial insemination

_____ 6. Zygote intrafallopian transfer

    a. Diagnosing conditions prior to a child's birth.

    b. Insertion of sperm into the woman's cervix by mechanical means.

    c. Removing a small amount of fluid from the amniotic sac.

    d. Eggs and sperm combined in laboratory and then inserted into fallopian tubes.

    e. Identifying possible disease through hereditary examination and review.

    f. Fertilization of the egg with the sperm occurs in a test tube.

## MULTIPLE-CHOICE QUESTIONS

_Instructions: Choose the one best answer for each question._

1. What is the study of ethical issues that result from technological and scientific advances?

   a. Biometrics

   b. Bioethics

   c. Biophysics

   d. Biogenesis

   (Objective 1)

2. Which of the following best describes biomedical ethics?

   a. A subdiscipline of a larger area of the philosophical study of morality

   b. Provides definitive answers about what is right and what is wrong in medical practice

   c. A discipline that has a long history

   d. Is fairly narrow in scope

   (Objective 1)

3. Which of the following represents what many believe to be the birth of bioethics?

   a. Establishment of the research center in Hastings, New York

   b. Recognition of the science through the establishment of a President's Commission

   c. Formal founding of the Kenney Institute Center for Bioethics

   d. Publication of an article in Life Magazine titled "They Decide Who Lives, Who Dies"

   (Objective 1)

4. Which of the following is responsible for creating many of our bioethical issues?

   a. The rising birth rate

   b. The rising death rate

   c. Technological advances

   d. The advent of psychopharmaceutics

   (Objective 1)

5. When were the first writings expressing concern about our growing population written?

   a. 1560

   b. 1600

   c. 1798

   d. 1850

   (Objective 2)

6. Which of the following represent one of the religious groups that forbid the use of artificial birth control?

   a. Jews

   b. Free Methodists

   c. Southern Baptists

   d. Roman Catholics

   (Objective 2)

7. Which of the following is an issue central to all discussions of contraception?

   a. The freedom to control one's body

   b. Greatest good for the greatest number

   c. The overpopulation of the world

   d. The rights of the unborn infant

   (Objective 2)

8. Which of the following is the major factor influencing how an individual may choose to practice contraception?

   a. A person' age

   b. A person's gender

   c. A person's heritage

   d. A person's values

   (Objective 2)

9. At one time it was believed that children could tell right from wrong and had reached the age of reason by which of the following ages?

   a. 5

   b. 7

   c. 10

   d. 15

   (Objective 2)

10. Under the concept of a mature minor, what must a minor do who wants access to birth control devices?

    a. First secure his or her parents' permission

    b. Demonstrate ability to pay for them

    c. Promise not to share them with friends

    d. Obtain them on request

    (Objective 2)

11. Which of the following represents the most liberal legislation as applied to the care of minors?

    a. Treatment of venereal disease

    b. Prescribing of birth control

    c. Birth of children

    d. Setting of broken bones

    (Objective 2)

12. Which group developed a Model Act in 1973, which addresses the issue of consent of minors for health care?

    a. Fellows of the College of OB/GYN

    b. Academy of Family Practitioners

    c. American Academy of Pediatrics

    d. American Psychiatric Association

    (Objective 2)

13. On what basis do conservatives argue against sex education and the dispensing of contraceptives by the schools?

    a. It is unsafe.

    b. It is immoral.

    c. It is too costly.

    d. It erodes the role of the family.

    (Objective 2)

14. To what does the age of consent refer?

    a. The age at which one may vote

    b. The age at which one may purchase alcoholic beverages

    c. The age at which one may witness legal documents

    d. The age at which one is capable of giving deliberate and voluntary agreement

    (Objective 2)

15. What is the term used to refer to an abortion that is done to save the life of the mother?

    a. Spontaneous

    b. Therapeutic

    c. Complete

    d. Elective

    (Objective 2)

16. Which of the following beliefs is central to people's concerns about the ethics of abortion?

    a. Life after death

    b. Passive euthanasia

    c. When life begins

    d. The value of life

    (Objective 2)

17. A decision by which one of the following groups resulted in legalized abortions in the United States in 1973?

    a. United States Supreme Court

    b. New York State Supreme Court

    c. Vatican

    d. Institute of Society, Ethics, and Life Sciences

    (Objective 2)

18. Which of the following is the concept on which we base the principle that it is wrong to give birth to a child whose life will not have the same quality as that of other children?

    a. Negative eugenics

    b. Wrongful birth

    c. Wrongful death

    d. Positive eugenics

    (Objective 2)

19. Which of the following is one of the arguments against programs of genetic screening?

    a. It is considered abnormal.

    b. It can lead to the downfall of a nation.

    c. It can place a great deal of strain on a marriage.

    d. It exceeds the bounds of what human beings should "tamper with."

    (Objective 3)

20. What is the term that refers to the science of improving the physical and mental qualities of human beings by controlling factors that influence heredity?

    a. Euthanasia

    b. Bioethics

    c. Cloning

    d. Eugenics

    (Objective 3)

21. What does negative eugenics advocate?

    a. Elimination of unwanted characteristics from a nation by discouraging "unworthy" parents from having children

    b. Increasing desirable traits in the population by urging "worthy" parents to have children

    c. Taking no extraordinary measures to sustain life

    d. Taking steps to hasten the individual's death

    (Objective 3)

22. What is the name applied to the project that has as one of its goals the detailed mapping of genetic makeup?

    a. Behavioral Response project

    b. Project Fifteen

    c. Genetic Determination Project

    d. Human Genome Project

    (Objective 3)

23. Which of the following is a goal of genetic research?

    a. Identify defective fetuses so that they could be aborted if the family wished

    b. Identify and isolate defective genes and replace them with functional genes

    c. Describe genetic makeup

    d. Provide a rationale for the practice of eugenics

    (Objective 3)

24. Which of the following refers to the practice by which a woman agrees to bear a child conceived through artificial insemination and to relinquish the baby at birth to others?

    a. In vitro fertilization

    b. Surrogate motherhood

    c. Adoption

    d. Family planning

    (Objective 4)

25. Which of the following represents a positive aspect of amniocentesis?

    a. It has heralded the development of prenatal surgery.

    b. It consistently results in more positive birthrates.

    c. It takes all the guesswork out of reproduction.

    d. It allows potential parents greater freedom of choice.

    (Objective 4)

26. Which of the following is a main reason couples request an amniocentesis?

    a. They want to know whether the child will be male or female.

    b. They are in an at-risk group.

    c. It is considered a desirable test for all mothers over 25.

    d. It will identify any congenital disease.

    (Objective 4)

27. Until recently, the most widely accepted definition of death was from which of the following?

    a. Old Testament

    b. United States Constitution

    c. Hippocratic Oath

    d. *Black's Law Dictionary*

    (Objective 5)

28. Newer definitions of death have been built around the concept of human potential. Which method is most often used to assess this capability?

    a. Computed tomography scan

    b. Electroencephalogram

    c. Electrocardiogram

    d. Magnetic resonance imaging

    (Objective 5)

29. For which of the following do we also use the definition of brain death?

    a. Seeking power of attorney

    b. Notifying next of kin

    c. Obtaining organs for transplantation

    d. Removing valuables

    (Objective 5)

30. Which one of the following statements is true of our definition of death?

    a. All parts of the body die simultaneously.

    b. The moment of death is unmistakable.

    c. The absence of brain waves over a given period of time is a generally accepted definition of death.

    d. Only after respirations have ceased for a period of 8 hours can the body be considered legally dead.

    (Objective 5)

31. Which of the following is true of a patient who has given informed consent?

    a. The patient totally accepts the plan of the treatment.

    b. The patient clearly understands the choices being offered.

    c. The patient participated in planning the treatment to be administered.

    d. The patient solicited a second opinion before signing papers.

    (Objective 7)

32. Which of the following has been cited as the basis for right-to-die issues?

    a. Fear of prolongation of dying due to medical intervention

    b. Fear of outliving one's children

    c. Fear that caring for too many elderly will bankrupt the nation

    d. Fear that there will not be enough facilities to meet the needs of everyone

    (Objective 7)

33. Which of the following is a critical issue when making decisions regarding withholding or withdrawing treatment?

    a. Whether the patient is legally competent

    b. Whether all papers granting power of attorney for health care have been completed

    c. Whether the patient has sufficient legal representation

    d. Whether all the family is in agreement

    (Objective 7)

34. Which of the following represents one of the major bioethical issues facing Americans today?

    a. Where to invest research dollars

    b. The feasibility of germ warfare

    c. The acquisition and allocation of scarce medical resources

    d. The rising cost of medical insurance

    (Objectives 8 and 10)

35. Which represents one of the problems highlighted by the need for donated organs?

    a. The cost of organ removal

    b. Identification of the gender of the person donating the organ

    c. Identification of the person who is responsible for approaching the family

    d. Whether the organ should be transported out of state

    (Objective 8)

36. Which of the following is cited as one reason organ donations from minority groups lag behind those of Caucasians?

    a. There is little demand for donated organs from among minority groups.

    b. The medical community prefers to use organs from Caucasians.

    c. There is not sufficient monetary reimbursement.

    d. Religious beliefs and cultural customs may forbid organ donation.

    (Objective 8)

37. What is the term used to refer to the practice of using animal organs, cells, and tissues for transplantation into human beings?

    a. Heterotransplantation

    b. Homotransplantation

    c. Somatransplantation

    d. Xenotransplantation

    (Objective 8)

38. Which of the following is a major consideration when applying ethical concerns to behavior control?

   a. Identifying what constitutes deviant behavior

   b. The age of consent

   c. The religious preference of the client

   d. The type of condition from which the client suffers

   (Objective 9)

39. Which type of behavior control is seldom used today?

   a. Administration of pharmacologic agents

   b. Electric shock therapy

   c. Electroconvulsive therapy

   d. Psychosurgery

   (Objective 9)

40. Of those listed below, which state has created a process by which health care priorities have been established?

   a. Arkansas

   b. Oregon

   c. Pennsylvania

   d. Texas

   (Objective 10)

# GAMING IN THE CLASSROOM

*Instructions: This game involves selecting teams and a host. The teams compete against one another for points. Each game has several subject categories. After teams are determined, a team is chosen to go first and selects a category. The host then poses the answer and the team provides the correct question for that answer. Each question can be awarded the same number of points or more difficult questions may be given heavier point values. (The instructor might determine which questions are more difficult based on the content emphasized in class.) Points are awarded to the team that is the first to signal and give a correct question. If that team is incorrect, the other team may attempt to provide the correct question and receive the points. The length of time allowed for response can be determined by the class or by the instructor. The team with the most points at the end of the game is declared the winner. Teams may be composed of individual students or groups of students. Teams may determine their answers as a team or may take turns answering as individuals.*

## Categories

A. Terms Used in Bioethics

B. Medical Milestones of the 1900s

C. Family Planning

D. Issues Related to Death

E. Withholding and Withdrawing Treatment

## Answers and Questions

### Category A

A:  A study of ethical issues that result from technological and scientific advances.

Q:  What is bioethics?

A:  The movement devoted to improving the human species through genetic control.

Q:  What is eugenics?

A:  All the genetic material in the chromosomes of a particular organism.

Q:  What is a genome?

A:  The identification and isolation of defective genes, and their replacement with functional genes.

Q:  What is gene therapy?

A:  The process by which an egg is fertilized in a test tube.

Q:  What is in vitro fertilization?

### Category B

A:  A disease that was declared eradicated worldwide 2 years after the last known case was identified.

Q: What is smallpox?

A: Doctors from New York and San Francisco first reported cases of this disease in 1979.

Q: What is acquired immunodeficiency syndrome (AIDS)?

A: This machine is able to assemble thousands of x-ray images into a highly detailed picture of the body.

Q: What is computer tomography (CAT)?

A: Represents the organ that is most successfully transplanted.

Q: What is the kidney?

A: Performed the first human heart transplant in 1967.

Q: Who is Christian Barnard?

## Category C

A: The right of an individual to obtain medical contraceptive advice was established through this court case.

Q: What is the case of *Griswold and Buxton v. the State of Connecticut*?

A: Encyclicals from this church forbid the use of artificial birth control.

Q: What is the Roman Catholic Church?

A: The age at which one is capable of giving deliberate and voluntary agreement.

Q: What is the age of consent?

A: A nurse who championed for contraceptive practices at a time when such activities were extremely unpopular.

Q: Who was Margaret Sanger?

A: An early essay that expressed deep concern about a population that was growing faster than were the resources to support it.

Q: What was "On Population"?

## Category D

A: Has traditionally provided us with the definition of death.

Q: What is *Black's Law Dictionary*?

A: The part of the body that dies most rapidly.

Q: What are brain cells?

A: Newer definitions of death are based around this concept.

Q: What is the concept of human potential?

A: Treatments that cannot, within a reasonable possibility, cure, ameliorate, improve, or restore a quality of life that would be satisfactory to the patient.

Q: What are futile treatments?

A: Requires that all Medicare and Medicaid providers inform patients on admission of their right to refuse treatment.

Q: What is the Patient Self-Determination Act?

## Category E

A: Refers to a situation in which no extraordinary or heroic measures are undertaken to sustain life.

Q: What is negative (or passive) euthanasia?

A: A landmark case related to the withdrawing of treatment.

Q: What was the case of Karen Quinlan?

A: A group that has issued a position statement of assisted suicide as it affects the practice of nursing.

Q: What is the American Nurses Association?

A: This organization developed a paper that provided clear definitions of key terms and a general guideline for making decisions regarding treatment.

Q: What is the Hastings Center?

A: This position paper stated that the decision to withhold medically provided nutrition and hydration should be made by the patient or surrogate with the health care team.

Q: What is the "Position Statement on Foregoing Medically Provided Nutrition and Hydration" published by the American Nurses Association?

# 11

# Beginning Your Career as a Nurse

## PURPOSE

This chapter helps the student to look toward employment as a nurse. Social changes affecting the new graduate, the various views of competency, and expectations of employers are discussed to assist students as they plan their own entry into the workforce. Suggestions for coping with expectations of others and for setting personal career goals are provided. Concrete directions are given for applying for a position, writing a résumé, and responding to an interview. The discussion of reality shock and burnout is designed to help the student prepare for these possibilities and approach them constructively.

## OBJECTIVES

1. Describe a variety of employment opportunities available to nurses today.

2. Explain the common competencies needed by the new graduate as outlined by the job analysis study.

3. Analyze the eight common expectations employers have of new graduates and relate them to your own background and education.

4. Develop a list of your personal short- and long-term career goals.

5. Describe how you plan to maintain your competence in nursing.

6. Create a personal résumé; sample letters of application, follow-up, and resignation; and a plan for your personal responses in an employment interview that can be used when you seek employment.

7. Explore strategies that you might personally use to prevent or alleviate reality shock.

8. Analyze your own values and life situation in relationship to your personal potential for burnout.

9. Discuss three areas of concern relative to sex discrimination in nursing.

10. Identify hazards to the health of both yourself and others in the nursing workplace and ways that you can act to protect yourself.

## KEY TERMS

| | |
|---|---|
| Burnout | Occupational hazard |
| Comparable worth | Reality shock |
| Competency | Résumé |
| Cover letter | Short-term goals |
| Long-term goals | Stereotype |
| Novice | |

## SITUATIONS TO FOSTER CRITICAL THINKING

1. Analyze your own background and identify your strengths and weaknesses. Develop an approach to presenting your strengths to a prospective employer and create a plan for your own growth.

2. In your clinical practice setting, identify the skills that nurses are currently using. Compare this with the common expectations outlined in the text and with what you know about other settings in your community.

3. Analyze the concept of reality shock and evaluate your own potential for experiencing this phenomenon. Do you believe that this is a problem to be avoided or a naturally occurring professional development phenomenon?

4. Set a short-term career goal and a long-term career goal. Identify the steps you will need to take to reach those goals.

5. There are few job opportunities for newly licensed registered nurses in your community. To conduct a successful job search, you will need to plan carefully. First, identify the various settings that might employ a new graduate in your community. Then outline the key skills and abilities you believe would be needed in each setting. Last, evaluate yourself in relationship to these key skills and abilities.

6. Develop a comprehensive list of questions that you believe might be asked in an employment interview for a registered nurse in your community. Plan personal answers to these questions.

## DISCUSSION/ESSAY QUESTIONS

1. What changes have occurred in the types of settings in which nurses are employed? (Objective 1)

2. What changes in hospitals have affected the roles of nurses in hospital settings? (Objective 1)

3. Identify a major change in the way health care is delivered and how this has affected the abilities of the new graduate. (Objective 2)

4. Identify a major change in the way nursing education is conducted and how this has affected the abilities of the new graduate. (Objective 2)

5. How has technology affected the role of the new graduate in nursing? (Objective 2)

6. Define competency as it applies to nursing and discuss how this will affect your practice as a beginning nurse. (Objective 2)

7. Compare the areas of competence that are of concern to employers with the nursing education you have received and evaluate yourself in relationship to these areas. (Objective 3)

8. Identify three of the consistent expectations that employers have of new graduates and discuss how you can act to meet those expectations. (Objective 3)

9. Identify one common area in which employers expect competence and discuss how you feel prepared to function in that area. (Objective 3)

10. Do you feel prepared to meet employers' expectations in regard to theoretical knowledge and use of the nursing process? Explain your answer. (Objective 3)

11. Two areas in which employers' expectations differ widely were mentioned. What is the situation in your geographical area in regard to these expectations? (Objective 3)

12. Briefly sketch a description of what you expect to be doing professionally 5, 10, and 20 years after graduation. (Objective 4)

13. What avenues are open to you to make yourself better prepared to meet employers' expectations? How might you go about using these? (Objective 5)

14. What should you include in a letter of application? (Objective 6)

15. What should you include in a résumé? (Objective 6)

16. What do you see as your greatest assets in an interview? Your greatest liabilities? (Objective 6)

17. Discuss how you might use an interview follow-up letter to increase your chances of obtaining a position you desire. (Objective 6)

18. Discuss ways in which you might tactfully indicate in a letter of resignation that you were leaving because the setting did not provide an opportunity for staff nurses to be involved in decision making about the delivery of nursing care. (Objective 6)

19. Define burnout and describe factors in nursing employment situations that might contribute to burnout. (Objective 8)

20. Identify specific actions you might take on your own behalf that could prevent reality shock. (Objective 7)

21. What factors in your own life might either help you avoid burnout or make you more susceptible to burnout? (Objective 8)

22. What specific actions can you take to prevent your own burnout? (Objective 8)

23. Discuss whether sex discrimination has affected the men enrolled in your nursing program. (Objective 9)

24. Identify actions that nurses could take to eliminate sex discrimination in nursing. (Objective 9)

25. Identify a hazard in the nursing workplace and measures you could take to avoid or minimize that hazard? (Objective 10)

26. Why is violence in the workplace a concern for nurses? (Objective 10)

## FILL IN THE BLANKS

*Instructions: Complete the following statements by filling in the blanks with the word or words that make the sentence complete and correct.*

1. Historically most nurses have been employed in _____. (Objective 1)

2. The growth of autonomy for nurses has been most evident _____ the hospital. (Objective 1)

3. The number of positions for nurses _____ ___ _____ have been growing. (Objective 1)

4. The number of men in nursing has been _____. (Objective 1)

5. The number of nurses employed outside of the hospital setting today is _____ than the past. (Objective 1)

6. The most definitive statement of competencies of the new graduate was identified by the _____. (Objective 2)

7. Competencies of the new graduates of various levels of nursing education have been developed by the _____ _____ of the NLN. (Objective 2)

8. The extent to which activities cannot be delayed or omitted with substantial risk of unnecessary complication, impairment of function, or serious distress to clients is called the activity's _____. (Objective 2)

9. Three consistent expectations that employers have of new graduates are _____ , _____ , and _____ . (Objective 2)

10. Knowledge of and appropriate use of _____ _____ as an infection control measure led the list of critically important nursing actions. (Objective 2)

11. The usual expectation of new graduates is that they use the following steps of the nursing process: _____, _____, _____, _____, and _____. (Objective 3)

12. To maintain safety, the new graduate must recognize his or her own _____ and _____. (Objective 3)

13. In addition to using communication skills with clients, the new graduate should be able to use them with _____. (Objective 3)

14. Getting to work on time, monitoring one's own breaks, and focusing on the job while at work is considered a commitment to a _____ _____. (Objective 3)

15. When planning personal career goals, you might include both clinical area and _____ area. (Objective 4)

16. Career goals are often focused on both a functional area and a _____ area. (Objective 4)

17. The first step in setting career goals is _____. (Objective 4)

18. Long-term goals represent where you wish to be in your profession _____ ____ _____ years from now. (Objective 4)

19. Maintaining continued competency is enhanced by _____ on the job. (Objective 5)

20. Courses designed to enhance continued competence are called _____ _____. (Objective 5)

21. A letter of resignation is usually sent _____ weeks before you will leave employment. (Objective 6)

22. Individuals who will attest to your abilities as an employee are termed _____. (Objective 6)

23. Your résumé should use _____ verbs. (Objective 6)

24. When considering jobs outside of health care, focus on the _____ you developed in each job. (Objective 6)

25. Reality shock is defined as _____ _____. (Objective 7)

26. One cause of reality shock is _____ expectations. (Objective 7)

27. Some less effective responses to reality shock are _____ and _____. (Objective 7)

28. To combat reality shock, the new graduate must be more _____ in regard to identifying professional needs. (Objective 7)

29. One approach to coping with reality shock is the technique of limiting the problems you will engage through the "politics of the _____." (Objective 7)

30. Burnout is a form of _____ _____. (Objective 8)

31. Symptoms of burnout include both _____ and _____. (Objective 8)

32. Prominent among causes of burnout is the conflict between _____ and _____. (Objective 8)

33. Burnout can best be prevented by mounting a stress-reduction effort by _____ _____, _____ _____, and _____ _____. (Objective 8)

34. _____ are sometimes the object of sex discrimination in nursing. (Objective 9)

35. Assigning similar salaries to occupations with similar education, skill level, and responsibilities is referred to as _____ _____. (Objective 9)

36. Behavior of a sexual nature that creates a work environment that is perceived as hostile and unduly stressful is termed _____ _____. (Objective 9)

37. The first step in stopping sexual harassment should be a _____ __ _____. (Objective 9)

38. Legal and ethical responsibility for providing a work environment free of sexual harassment is the responsibility of the _____. (Objective 9)

39. The first step in controlling hazards in the workplace is _____ _____. (Objective 10)

40. Gloves cannot prevent the transmission of blood-borne infections that occur from _____ _____. (Objective 10)

41. The precautions recommended by the CDC to provide maximum protection from infection for health care workers are _____ _____. (Objective 10)

42. Two-thirds of nonfatal workplace assaults occur in _____ and _____ _____ agencies. (Objective 10)

43. OSHA guidelines on violence in the workplace recommend that there be an _____ and _____ of problems and a _____ for prevention. (Objective 10)

# TRUE-FALSE QUESTIONS

*Instructions: Mark the following statements "T" if true or "F" if false. If using a scoring card, mark "A" if true or "B" if false.*

_____ 1. In the early part of the 20th century, most nurses were employed by hospitals. (Objective 1)

_____ 2. The 1930s saw a change in nursing in that nurses were no longer expected to be "on duty" for an entire 24-hour period. (Objective 1)

_____ 3. One change in nursing created by World War II was the employment of married nurses. (Objective 1)

_____ 4. In the 1940s, most graduates of hospital schools of nursing were employed by the hospitals in which they received their education. (Objective 1)

_____ 5. Competency refers to the ability to perform as expected. (Objective 2)

_____ 6. Changes in nursing education in the last 20 years have resulted in not every student having an opportunity to perform every skill. (Objective 2)

_____ 7. There is no general consensus whatever regarding essential competence for new nurse graduates. (Objective 2)

_____ 8. Ability to recognize one's own abilities and limitations is considered an essential competency in every setting. (Objective 2)

_____ 9. Employers are generally concerned with the new nurse's ability to use technical skills. (Objective 3)

_____ 10. Employers generally expect that they will have to teach the nursing process to new nurses. (Objective 3)

_____ 11. Employers generally expect new nurses to know their own strengths and weaknesses and to ask for help. (Objective 3)

_____ 12. Employers generally do not expect that new nurses will understand the demands of record keeping. (Objective 3)

_____ 13. There are wide differences in the degree of technical skill that employers expect of new nurses. (Objective 3)

_____ 14. There is general agreement about the speed at which new nurses are expected to function. (Objective 3)

_____ 15. For the new graduate, personal career goals should focus only on the short term. (Objective 4)

_____ 16. Personal career goals may include a focus on a clinical area. (Objective 4)

_____ 17. Personal career goals may include a focus on a functional area. (Objective 4)

_____ 18. Long-term goals should represent where a person wants to be by the end of his or her career. (Objective 4)

_____ 19. Continuing education is legally required of nurses in every setting. (Objective 5)

_____ 20. On-the-job learning is considered a valid way to maintain continued competence. (Objective 5)

_____ 21. Every nurse if obligated to maintain competence. (Objective 5)

_____ 22. A letter of application should include an overview of the applicant's qualifications for the position being sought. (Objective 6)

_____ 23. A résumé should include reference to special honors or recognition received while a nursing student. (Objective 6)

_____ 24. A résumé should include offices held in social organizations. (Objective 6)

_____ 25. It is inappropriate to ask questions regarding salary and benefits in an interview. (Objective 6)

_____ 26. Employers are free to ask any question they wish of applicants. (Objective 6)

_____ 27. It is appropriate to ask questions regarding policies and procedures during an interview. (Objective 6)

_____ 28. After an interview, you should wait for the employer to contact you. (Objective 6)

_____ 29. An interview follow-up letter includes a reference to any agreements or commitments made by the employer during the interview. (Objective 6)

_____ 30. If you have been unhappy in a job, the letter of resignation is the best place to inform your employer of your grievances. (Objective 6)

_____ 31. A formal letter of resignation is necessary only if you have a management position. (Objective 6)

_____ 32. A letter of resignation is often sent to more than one person in the organization. (Objective 6)

_____ 33. Reality shock refers to feelings that result from encountering a more complex and difficult work situation than expected and feeling powerless to affect the situation. (Objective 7)

_____ 34. An externship is a program to help nursing students become more familiar and comfortable with the employment setting while they are still students. (Objective 7)

_____ 35. Reality shock may be a realistic part of the passage from novice to experienced nurse. (Objective 7)

_____ 36. One result of reality shock is "job hopping." (Objective 7)

_____ 37. Burnout is more likely to happen in units that have inadequate staffing. (Objective 8)

_____ 38. Burnout occurs only in those who have underlying mental health problems. (Objective 8)

_____ 39. Burnout decreases problem-solving capabilities. (Objective 8)

_____ 40. Burnout can be prevented by a focused effort in stress reduction. (Objective 8)

_____ 41. Unlike women in a man's field, men in nursing are not subject to sex discrimination. (Objective 9)

_____ 42. Comparable worth is a concept accepted by most health care employers. (Objective 9)

_____ 43. Sexual harassment usually represents an exercise of power over others. (Objective 9)

_____ 44. Employers are responsible for the working environment. (Objective 9)

_____ 45. The transmission of infection is considered a workplace hazard for nurses. (Objective 10)

_____ 46. Standard precautions (body substance precautions) are mandated by OSHA regulation. (Objective 10)

_____ 47. Violence is a workplace concern for nurses. (Objective 10)

_____ 48. The highest incidence in health care setting of work-related back injuries is among nursing assistants. (Objective 10)

## MULTIPLE-CHOICE QUESTIONS

_Instructions: Choose the one best answer for each question._

1. Which of the following has historically been the setting in which most new graduates were employed?

   a. Hospital

   b. Health-related businesses

   c. Outpatient setting

   d. Community nursing agency

   (Objective 1)

2. Historically where did most education for nursing students occur?

   a. Hospital

   b. Health-related businesses

   c. Outpatient setting

   d. Community nursing agency

   (Objective 1)

3. What is the fastest growing area of employment for nurses?

   a. Hospitals

   b. Health-related businesses

   c. Surgery centers

   d. Community nursing settings

   (Objective 1)

4. What has been characteristic of non-hospital settings for nurses?

   a. Increased autonomy

   b. More constraints on practice

   c. The failure to use nursing skills appropriately

   d. The limited use of the multi-disciplinary team

   (Objective 1)

5. Which of the following has decreased the new graduate's ability to perform according to the hospital's procedures?

   a. New graduates do not learn procedures anymore.

   b. Individuals are not necessarily employed in institutions where they had education experiences.

   c. Most new nurses have less education than previously.

   d. The focus of nursing education is on outpatient care, not hospital care.

   (Objective 2)

6. Recently nursing organizations and groups have looked at various educational paths to nursing education to define what those who follow each should be able to do. What are these abilities called?

   a. Outcome behaviors

   b. Competencies

   c. Levels of performance

   d. Skills

   (Objective 2)

7. What is competence?

   a. Ability to work independently

   b. Ability to meet the minimum standards of the job

   c. Ability to perform with expert skill

   d. Ability to compete with others for a job

   (Objective 3)

8. The most widely accepted definition of competence has been established by the

   a. National League for Nursing

   b. National Council of State Boards of Nursing

   c. American Nurses Association

   d. American Association of Colleges of Nursing

   (Objective 3)

9. What do employers want new graduates to have?

   a. The necessary theoretical background for basic patient care and decision making

   b. The ability to function efficiently within one week of assuming a new position

   c. Little need for supervision after the first month

   d. An understanding of hospital policies

   (Objective 3)

10. Which of the following is an expectation that employers consistently have of new employees?

    a. That they perform all technical skills without assistance

    b. That they are comfortable with hospital policy

    c. That they will recognize their own abilities and limitations

    d. That they will be able to assume charge of the unit in 6 months

    (Objective 3)

11. What is expected of the new graduate in regard to record keeping?

    a. Records should be completed independently.

    b. The new graduate will not be responsible for records.

    c. The ability to use computerized records is expected.

    d. The new graduate must know what must be recorded.

    (Objective 3)

12. Which of the following do most employers expect of new graduates?

    a. Skill in carrying out procedures

    b. Efficiency in carrying out responsibilities

    c. Ability to use the nursing process effectively

    d. Proficiency in the charting system in use

    (Objective 3)

13. In which of the following may expectations of the new graduate vary widely?

    a. In different facilities and in different geographical areas

    b. From one graduate of the program to another

    c. From one class to another

    d. Within the same geographical area

    (Objective 3)

14. Which of the following is the least effective method of coping with expectations of the employer?

    a. Review your own abilities before graduation and seek experiences.

    b. Look for employment only in a facility where you practiced as a student.

    c. Seek an employer with an orientation program that matches your needs.

    d. Start a support group with other new graduates.

    (Objective 3)

15. What is the recommended first step in setting your personal goals?

    a. Review the clinical evaluation done while you were a student

    b. Ask your friends what they think you would do the best

    c. Do a thorough self-assessment

    d. Determine which areas of the hospital need your help the most

    (Objective 4)

16. When planning for career goals, what should you include?

    a. A clinical focus only

    b. A functional focus only

    c. A personal focus only

    d. Both a clinical and a functional focus

    (Objective 4)

17. Long-term goals are usually considered those that reflect where you want to be in your career in which of the following?

    a. 1 year

    b. 3 to 5 years

    c. 5 to 10 years

d. 20 to 30 years

(Objective 4)

18. Which of the following are useful ways to maintain competence in nursing?

a. Attend continuing education

b. Learn on the job

c. Read journals

d. All of the above

(Objective 5)

19. To maintain competence in nursing, some states require that you do which of the following?

a. Attend continuing education

b. Learn on the job

c. Read journals

d. All of the above

(Objective 5)

20. What is the best length for a résumé for a new graduate?

a. One page

b. Two pages

c. Three pages

d. Four pages

(Objective 6)

21. Which of the following should you do to prepare for an interview?

a. Outline questions you will want to ask

b. Be as casual as possible

c. Consider canceling the interview and rescheduling later if are you too nervous

d. Purchase a new suit so you will look professional

(Objective 6)

22. Which of the following is the most critical in an interview?

a. Be neat and well groomed

b. Have a good understanding of the philosophy of the hospital

c. Do not act nervous

d. Limit comments to the answers to questions posed by the interviewer

(Objective 6)

23. Which of the following is essential to presenting yourself effectively in an interview for a beginning nursing position?

a. Have your hair done professionally

b. Take a class on interviewing techniques

c. Purchase new "businesslike" clothing

d. Reflect on your personal philosophy of nursing

(Objective 6)

24. What is a major purpose of an interview follow-up letter?

a. Add information you forgot to give in your interview

b. Ask additional questions about the organization

c. Restate any agreements that were reached

d. Review important points you made during the interview

(Objective 6)

25. To whom should a letter of resignation be directed?

a. The hospital administrator

b. The nursing administrator

c. The personnel department

d. Your shift charge nurse

(Objective 6)

26. What is the situation in which the new graduate becomes frustrated because it may seem impossible to deliver quality care under the constraints in force?

    a. Disassociation

    b. Reality shock

    c. Displacement

    d. Burnout

    (Objective 7)

27. Which of the following is a program designed to provide a planned, organized transition period in which the new graduate participates in classes, seminars, and rotations to various units of the hospital?

    a. On-the-job training

    b. Orientation

    c. Externship

    d. Internship

    (Objective 7)

28. Which is true of reality shock?

    a. It represents a severe emotional problem requiring mental health care.

    b. It reflects inadequate basic preparation for the nursing role.

    c. It may be a realistic transition in the path from novice to experienced nurse.

    d. It requires that institutions make major changes in order to prevent.

    (Objective 7)

29. What is one of the common effects of reality shock?

    a. Giving up ideals of nursing practice

    b. Emotional breakdown

    c. Renewed impetus to improve one's own practice

    d. Joining together with others to improve the situation

    (Objective 7)

30. Which of the following is a personal strategy that might effectively combat burnout without jeopardizing your career?

    a. Decrease your physical exercise to conserve energy

    b. Plan for a group of nurses to share concerns

    c. Stay no longer than one year in a position

    d. Take extra vitamins

    (Objective 8)

31. Symptoms of burnout are related to which of the following?

    a. G.I. disorders

    b. Muscle tension

    c. Fatigue

    d. Chronic stress

    (Objective 8)

32. Symptoms of burnout include which of the following?

    a. Physical changes

    b. Psychological difficulties

    c. Interpersonal difficulties

    d. All of the above

    (Objective 8)

33. What is an area of recent economic concern in nursing?

    a. Comparable worth

    b. Nepotism

    c. Civil rights

    d. Shift differentials

    (Objective 9)

34. Which employment area in nursing has sometimes been discriminatory toward men?

    a. Long-term care

b. Obstetrics

c. Pediatrics

d. Surgery

(Objective 9)

35. What is sexual harassment?

    a. Not a concern in health care environments

    b. So vague a term as to be useless in nursing

    c. Primarily related to sexual feelings

    d. A demonstration of personal power over another person

    (Objective 9)

36. Employers may be required to provide immunization for employees who have significant risk for which of the following?

    a. AIDS

    b. Tetanus

    c. Hepatitis B

    d. Tuberculosis

    (Objective 10)

37. Nurses have a high incidence of which of the following work-related problems?

    a. Falls

    b. Back injuries

    c. Skin damage

    d. Infections

    (Objective 10)

38. What does OSHA mandate that employers provide?

    a. Universal precautions supplies

    b. Standard precautions supplies

    c. Mechanical lifting equipment

    d. Needless intravenous access devices

    (Objective 10)

39. According to OSHA, in what employment setting do the most incidents of violence against workers occur?

    a. Retail sales establishments

    b. Jails

    c. Prisons

    d. Health and social service agencies

    (Objective 10)

40. Which of the following work-related hazards is present in almost every area of nursing?

    a. Anesthetic gases

    b. AIDS

    c. Chemotherapeutic agents

    d. Toxic chemicals

    (Objective 10)

## GAMING IN THE CLASSROOM

*Instructions: This game involves selecting teams and a host. The teams compete against one another for points. Each game has several subject categories. After teams are determined, a team is chosen to go first and selects a category. The host then poses the answer and the team provides the correct question for that answer. Each question can be awarded the same number of points or more difficult questions may be given heavier point values. (The instructor might determine which questions are more difficult based on the content emphasized in class.) Points are awarded to the team that is the first to signal and give a correct question. If that team is incorrect, the other team may attempt to provide the correct question and receive the points. The length of time allowed for response can be determined by the class or by the instructor. The team with the most points at the end of the game is declared the winner. Teams may be composed of individual students or groups of students. Teams may determine their answers as a team or may take turns answering as individuals.*

## Categories

A. Competency for New Graduates

B. Job Seeking

C. Job-Stress Concerns

D. Sex Discrimination in Nursing

## Answers and Questions

### Category A

A: Competencies separated for each type of RN education.

Q: What kind of competencies were written by the educational councils of the NLN?

A: A complex research study of new graduates.

Q: How were the competencies for the NLCEX-RN developed?

A: Criticality of each action.

Q: What was a key criterion by which each nursing activity was judged in the NLCEX-RN research study?

A: A work ethic.

Q: What do employers expect?

A: Technical skill competency.

Q: Which area of competency has the greatest variability in expectation?

### Category B

A: Résumé.

Q: What is a one-page summary of ones' job qualifications called?

A: Letter of application (cover letter).

Q: How should you address requirements of a specific job announcement when applying?

A: Names, addresses, permission.

Q: What information do you need about references before using them?

A: Action-oriented verbs.

Q: What is the preferred style for writing job responsibilities in a résumé?

A: Role-playing.

Q: What is an effective way to prepare for a job interview?

A: "How old are you?"

Q: What is it illegal to ask in an employment interview?

### Category C

A: Reality shock.

Q: What is the job-stress syndrome that occurs in new RNs called?

A: Burnout.

Q: What is the term for chronic job-related stress?

A: Personal experience and personal knowing.

Q: What is the basis for expert practice?

A: Unrealistic expectations of self.

Q: What is a cause of reality shock?

A: Self-assessment.

Q: What is the first step in preventing job-related stress?

### Category D

A: Obstetrical units.

Q: Where has sex discrimination against men in nursing been identified?

A: American Assembly for Men in Nursing.

Q: What organization has as its purpose equitable practice opportunities for men in nursing?

A: A demonstration of personal power over others.

Q: What is the foundation of sexual harassment?

A: Employer.

Q: Who has the responsibility for maintaining a working environment free of sex discrimination?

A: Tell the individual the behavior is unwanted and unacceptable.

Q: What should be the first response to behavior that reflects sexual harassment?

# 12

# Preparing for Workplace Participation

## PURPOSE

This chapter presents information basic to assuming a staff nurse role in the health care delivery system. Material regarding the organizational structure of institutions is discussed followed by a review of the various patterns of nursing care delivery. The basic activities related to collective bargaining are explored, and the language used in collective bargaining is explained. Starting with a history of collective bargaining, the rules governing labor relations are discussed. The chapter considers the issues that arise with collective bargaining in the nursing profession and examines what to look for in a contract. The chapter concludes with a discussion of the grievance process and why it should be included in the contract.

## OBJECTIVES

1. Discuss the purpose of mission statements.

2. Analyze the relationships among organizational charts, chains of command, and channels of communication within organizations.

3. Delineate the characteristics of shared governance and the advantages of a shared governance approach.

4. Describe various patterns of nursing care delivery, identifying the major characteristics of each.

5. Discuss the history of collective bargaining as it applies to nursing.

6. Analyze the processes through which resolution is achieved in collective bargaining issues.

7. Identify at least four professional concerns that should be addressed in a contract for nurses.

8. Discuss the concerns nurses have regarding membership in a collective bargaining group and the reasons for these concerns.

9. Outline the advantages and disadvantages of having the state nurses' association serve as a bargaining agent for nurses.

10. Compare and contrast the characteristics of a grievance and a complaint.

## KEY TERMS

Accountability
Agency shop
Authoritative mandate
Authority
Bargain in good faith
Binding arbitration
Broad span of control
Case method
Chain of command
Channels of communication
Clinical ladder
Collective action division
Collective bargaining
Common interest bargaining
Concession bargaining
Contract
Cross-training
Deadlock
Division of labor
Final offer
Flat organization
Functional method
Government seizure

Grievance process
Impasse
Informational picketing
Injunction
Job description
Lockout
Mediation
Mission statement
Narrow span of control
National Labor Relations Act
National Labor Relations Board
Negotiate/negotiation
Organization
Organizational chart
Organizational hierarchy
Policy
Professional collectivism
Protocol
Ratify
Reinstatement privilege
Role transition
Shared governance
Span of control

Standards of care      Unfair labor practice
Tall organization      Union busting
Team nursing           Unions
Total patient care

## SITUATIONS TO FOSTER CRITICAL THINKING

1. Review copies of the mission statement for the college you are attending and at least one of the health care facilities to which you are assigned for clinical experience. What do the statements have in common? How are they different? Do they speak to the purpose of each organization? Do they incorporate a statement of philosophy or are those separate statements? How would you change them?

2. You are working as a new graduate on the medical unit of a community hospital. You believe that there is a more efficient way to assign breaks and rotate off the unit for lunch. How would you go about sharing your plan and working toward its successful implementation? What steps would you take if your plan was rejected although you still believed it would be more effective than the system currently being used?

3. You are employed in an acute care hospital and have been informed that the pattern of care delivery is to be changed from primary nursing to a modular approach to care in which each module will have one registered nurse and two other care providers. These two additional care providers may be licensed practical nurses, nursing students, or nursing assistants. What are the skills you will need in this new pattern of care delivery that you did not need in the original pattern? What concerns will you have about this new pattern of care delivery? What questions do you need to ask to plan for the transition? What are the benefits and the drawbacks to this new plan?

4. You have identified that the system for recording medication administration in the subacute care unit where you work requires that p.r.n. medications be recorded in three different places and that frequently one of these is omitted by the nurses. This causes confusion and you find yourself spending excessive time checking and double-checking. How might you seek to change this procedure? Consider the lines of authority and accountability and roles of various individuals as you plan. What information do you need before you take any action?

5. Identify the patterns of care delivery that are being used in the hospitals in which you have received your clinical experience. Compare and contrast those care patterns. Why do you think each was chosen by the facility that is using it? From your perspective, which system is most effective and efficient? Why do you believe this is true? What differences do you see in the role of the registered nurse in each of these settings? What different skills does each pattern require of the nurse?

6. Consider that you are working in an acute care hospital that is covered by a collective bargaining contract and the administration decides to restructure the organization. Is this proposal related to rights under the contract? What information do you need to gather to determine this? Which individuals should be involved in decision making regarding the proposed restructuring?

7. Mary Watkins, RN, works in a hospital that has a policy of placing nurses on probation if they have three medication errors. She notes that many nurses do not fill out quality assurance (QA) reports when medication errors occur; however, she has always been very careful to follow the policy and complete QA reports. She makes a third error and is notified that she is being placed on probation. Would this be grievable under a contract? What questions would she need to ask to determine this? What considerations do

you think have a bearing on this case? What would you do if you were in this situation?

8. Jim Nathan, RN, works in a long-term care facility. The nursing assistants are considering establishing a union to bargain with the corporation that owns the facility. Would Jim be part of their union? What should be his role in the process? What degree of support do you believe he should provide to the nursing assistants? Why? Provide a rationale for the actions you think he should take.

## DISCUSSION/ESSAY QUESTIONS

1. Review the mission statement for your college. Does it speak to the purpose of the organization? Can you see where your program fits within that statement? (Objective 1)

2. Identify the mission statement or statement of purpose and philosophy of a local health care agency. Analyze how this statement affects the type of service offered. (Objective 1)

3. Compare and contrast the mission statement of a local hospital with that of a community-based health care facility. Are there similarities? Are there differences? What are they? (Objective 1)

4. Obtain a copy of the philosophy of the nursing care in the hospital to which you are assigned. What statements does it include that you expected to be there? What did it state that surprised you? (Objective 1)

5. Compare the organization of your college, a local hospital, and a long-term care facility in your community. How are they similar? How are they different? (Objective 2)

6. Examine the organizational chart of a local health care agency. What is the title of the highest level administrator? Who reports to that individual? (Objective 2)

7. Discuss the relationship among organizational charts, chains of command, and channels of communication. (Objective 2)

8. Make a chart of the reporting relationships on a unit of the hospital where you have practiced as a student. Be sure to include all the positions on the unit including those not filled by nurses. (Objective 2)

9. Is the hospital where you had your most recent clinical experience designed with a tall organizational structure or a flat one? What leads you to this conclusion? (Objective 2)

10. Analyze the organizational structure of one of the community-based organizations to which you have been assigned for clinical experience. How does that agency's structure differ from the structure of the hospital to which you were assigned? (Objective 2)

11. Look for job descriptions for the various positions in the hospital to which you are assigned for clinical experience. Where did you find those job descriptions? (Objective 2)

12. Look at the governance structure of a local hospital. How would you describe it? (Objective 3)

13. Look at the governance structure of a local long-term care facility. How would you describe it? (Objective 3)

14. Review the policy manual on the unit to which you are assigned for clinical experience. What items are covered in the manual? Where on the unit is that manual kept? (Objectives 2 and 3)

15. How are procedures updated or changed in the hospital to which you are assigned for clinical experience? (Objective 3)

16. How does the staff nurse on a unit in the hospital to which you are assigned for clinical experience have input into the hospital governance structure? (Objective 3)

17. Compare and contrast primary, team, and functional nursing. (Objective 4)

18. Analyze the patterns of nursing care delivery of health care facilities in which you have worked as a student. Why do you believe each type was used where it was? (Objective 4)

19. Which pattern of nursing care delivery do you believe to be the best and why? (Objective 4)

20. Discuss the role of the case manager in today's health care delivery system. (Objective 4)

21. Discuss what is meant by the term *negotiate*. (Objective 5)

22. Briefly outline the history of collective bargaining. (Objective 5)

23. In general, what is the role of the National Labor Relations Board (NLRB)? (Objective 5)

24. Why was it once seen as incongruous with values of nursing for nurses to negotiate salaries? Why has that changed? (Objective 5)

25. Why were nurses among the last of the professions to be included in national labor laws? (Objective 5)

26. What factors have made it difficult for nurses to bargain collectively for salaries? Which of these do you believe had the greatest influence and why? (Objective 5)

27. What exceptions to the national laws were made when nurses were included in the laws? Why was it thought that these were necessary? (Objective 5)

28. Define the terms *union, mediate,* and *arbitrate*. (Objective 6)

29. Define the term *collective action division*. (Objective 6)

30. Discuss several activities that could be considered unfair labor practices. (Objective 6)

31. What is the purpose of negotiating an agency shop? (Objective 6)

32. Discuss the role of the mediator and the arbitrator in a collective bargaining situation. (Objective 6)

33. Discuss at least two types of arbitration, explaining how they differ. (Objective 6)

34. What is a contract and why is it desirable to have one? (Objective 7)

35. List at least three items that should be included in a nurse's contract. (Objective 7)

36. What concerns do most nurses have when a strike is called? (Objective 7)

37. What are some arguments supporting strike activities by nurses? (Objective 7)

38. What provisions should be made to continue care of the community if a strike is called? Do you think there should be these provisions? (Objective 7)

39. Why does the role of the supervisor present problems to nurses from a collective bargaining viewpoint? (Objective 8)

40. Discuss the issues of professionalism versus unionism in nursing. Do you believe it is an issue that is no longer important? (Objective 8)

41. Why are nurses sometimes reluctant to join a bargaining group? (Objective 8)

42. Give some reasons why many nurses believe they are best represented at the bargaining table by the state nurses' association. (Objective 9)

43. Are there reasons why nurses might be better represented at the bargaining table by another group? What problems might this create? (Objective 9)

44. Explain the purpose of a grievance process. (Objective 10)

45. How does a grievance differ from a complaint? (Objective 10)

# FILL IN THE BLANKS

*Instructions: Complete the following statements by filling in the blanks with the word or words that make the sentence complete and correct.*

1. The statement that indicates the broad aims of a hospital is called its _____ _____. (Objective 1)

2. Breaking work into pieces or tasks that are assigned to various individuals or groups is known as _____ ___ _____. (Objective 2)

3. The graphic, pictorial means of portraying various roles and patterns of interaction among parts of a system is called the _____ _____. (Objective 2)

4. When discussing the number of employees supervised by a manager, we are talking about the _____ __ _____. (Objective 2)

5. The path of authority and accountability from individuals at the top of the organization to those at the base of the organization is known as the _____ __ _____. (Objective 2)

6. The patterns of message-giving within organizations is known as the _____ __ _____. (Objective 2)

7. The distribution and acceptance of a task or job or the obligation to take on and accomplish an assignment is referred to as _____. (Objective 2)

8. Written statements that describe the duties and functions of the various jobs within the organization are called ____ _____. (Objective 2)

9. When we teach one member of the health care team to perform functions usually associated with another position, it is known as _____ _____. (Objective 2)

10. A mechanism for recognizing and rewarding nurses who wish to remain in direct care positions rather than seek administrative positions is the _____ _____. (Objectives 2 and 3)

11. The document that spells out how a particular nursing activity is to be completed is known as the _____ _____. (Objectives 2 and 3)

12. Authoritive statements that describe a common or acceptable level of client care or performance are known as _____ __ _____. (Objective 2)

13. A structure that allows nursing staff to make major decisions within the organization is the _____ _____ structure. (Objective 3)

14. The shared governance format may take a number of approaches, such as the _____ model, the _____ model, or the _____ model. (Objective 3)

15. The _____ _____ was the first system used for the delivery of nursing care in the United States. (Objective 4)

16. When one nurse does all the temperatures, and another administers all the medications, while yet another does all the treatments, the unit is employing a _____ _____ of care delivery. (Objective 4)

17. When members of a nursing team come together to communicate about the needs of their patients and to plan for care, it is known as a _____ _____. (Objective 4)

18. Conferences among those who are providing care to a group of patients are essential to the functioning of _____ nursing. (Objective 4)

19. When one is responsible for initiating and updating the nursing care plan, patient teaching, and discharge planning and is assigned the responsibility for care of the patient from time of admission to discharge, one is working as a _____ nurse. (Objective 4)

20. The process of monitoring an individual patient's health care for the purpose of maximizing positive outcomes and

containing costs is _____ _____. (Objective 4)

21. The process of assigning a competent individual the responsibility of performing a particular nursing task in a selected situation is _____. (Objective 4)

22. Bargaining or conferring with another party or parties to reach an agreement is called _____. (Objective 5)

23. In the year _____, amendments to the National Labor Relations Act (NLRA) made it possible for employees of non-profit health care institutions to bargain collectively. (Objective 5)

24. What party will represent a group at the bargaining table is determined by _____. (Objective 5)

25. An early reformer who generated interest in collective bargaining was _____ _____. (Objective 5)

26. The NLRA passed in 1935 was also known as the _____. (Objective 5)

27. In 1947, the original labor act was amended through the _____ _____, which was also known as the _____ _____ _____ _____. (Objective 5)

28. The process by which the employer and employee representatives begin by identifying those areas in which they agree and those goals or values held by both parties is called _____ _____ _____. (Objective 5)

29. When a branch of a professional association assumes the responsibility of negotiating contracts for its members, the negotiating group may be known as a (an) _____ _____ _____. (Objectives 5 and 6)

30. A (An) _____ _____ _____ is any action that interferes with the rights of employees or employers as described in the amended NLRA. (Objective 5)

31. The advantage to a union of having a contract with an agency shop clause is that it _____ _____ _____ _____ _____. (Objective 5)

32. In _____ _____, both parties are obligated to abide by the decision of the arbitrator. (Objective 6)

33. When the parties doing the negotiating cannot come to an agreement on an issue, they are said to be at an _____ or the two groups are _____ on the issue. (Objective 6)

34. A major criticism of the arbitration process is_____. (Objective 6)

35. Three items that should be included in a contract for nurses are _____ _____, _____ _____, and _____ _____ _____. (Objective 7)

36. The organizations that have carried out the majority of the collective bargaining activities for nurses are the _____. (Objective 7)

37. When the negotiation process does not go smoothly, the last alternative available to the employee is to _____. (Objective 8)

38. Organized nurses in some states have focused their bargaining energies on issues of _____ _____. (Objective 9)

39. The grievance process spells out in _____ a series of steps to be taken to _____ the area of dissension. (Objective 10)

40. A (An) _____ is an allegation by any party functioning under a collective bargaining agreement that a violation of the contract has occurred. (Objective 10)

## TRUE-FALSE QUESTIONS

*Instructions: Mark the following statements "T" if true or "F" if false. If using a scoring card, mark "A" if true or "B" if false.*

_____ 1. The mission statement usually identifies the general purposes of the organization. (Objective 1)

_____ 2. The mission statement and accompanying philosophy have little to do with the evaluation of the organization's performance. (Objective 1)

_____ 3. Health care delivery organizations are usually considered bureaucratic organizations because they are operated and administered through a number of departments and subdivisions. (Objective 2)

_____ 4. In organizational theory, the concept of management is associated with the financial balance sheet for the institution. (Objective 2)

_____ 5. The organizational chart is typically represented by boxes stacked in a pyramid-shaped chart. (Objective 2)

_____ 6. In a flat organizational structure, the supervisor usually has a narrow span of control. (Objective 2)

_____ 7. Today, most health care organizations are moving toward a broader span of control. (Objective 2)

_____ 8. The chain of command represents the patterns of message-giving within an organization. (Objective 2)

_____ 9. Accountability involves a liability factor and can be defined as the liability for task performance. (Objective 2)

_____ 10. Job descriptions define the duties and functions of the various jobs within the organization but not the scope of authority, responsibility, or accountability. (Objective 2)

_____ 11. When a respiratory therapist is taught to perform some basic nursing care functions, it is an example of cross-training. (Objective 2)

_____ 12. A policy is a designated plan or course of action for a specific situation. (Objective 2)

_____ 13. Standards of care spell out how a particular nursing activity is to be completed, often describing the number of steps. (Objective 2)

_____ 14. Standards for patient care have been defined by the National League for Nursing and are widely distributed. (Objective 2)

_____ 15. Shared governance is a form of a professional practice model that involves shared decision making by nursing staff and nursing management. (Objective 3)

_____ 16. The implementation of shared governance models requires that staff nurses participate in professional development sessions that increase nurses' understanding of the decision-making process, team building, group dynamics, leadership, and budgeting. (Objective 3)

_____ 17. In a total patient care method of assignment, the nurse has responsibility for planning and supervising the individual patient's care for 24 hours a day. (Objective 4)

_____ 18. The situation in which we are most likely to see the case method of nursing care delivery today is in home health care. (Objective 4)

_____ 19. All case managers are registered nurses with a baccalaureate degree. (Objective 4)

_____ 20. All case managers follow patients from before admission, throughout hospitalization, and until they are discharged from home care. (Objective 4)

_____ 21. As early as 1850, reformers were interested in collective bargaining issues. (Objective 5)

_____ 22. The Wagner Act made it possible for nurses to bargain collectively for salaries. (Objective 2)

_____ 23. The role of the NLRB is to ensure that the conditions of labor legislation are properly enforced. (Objective 5)

_____ 24. The NLRA has never been amended. (Objective 5)

_____ 25. Collective action divisions operate under different constraints than do unions. (Objective 5)

_____ 26. The issue of agency shop is one rather frequently agreed on in the negotiation process. (Objective 5)

_____ 27. If a contract is *ratified*, it has been accepted by the members of the bargaining group. (Objective 5)

_____ 28. A mediator may never serve as an arbitrator. (Objective 6)

_____ 29. The final offer approach is a type of binding arbitration. (Objective 6)

_____ 30. A lockout is said to occur when an employer closes a factory or other place of business to make employees agree to terms. (Objectives 5 and 6)

_____ 31. A mediator is a third person who may join the bargainers to assist in the reconciliation of differences. (Objective 6)

_____ 32. Binding arbitration means that both parties are obligated to abide by the decision of the arbitrator. (Objective 6)

_____ 33. There are no specific criteria for the content to be included in a contract. (Objective 7)

_____ 34. In the collective bargaining process, supervisors function just as any other member of the employees' group. (Objective 7)

_____ 35. Federal law makes it illegal for nurses to strike. (Objective 8)

_____ 36. The right to bargain collectively was initially a controversial issue among nurses and other members of the health care team. (Objective 8)

_____ 37. A definition of the collective professional role should not be a part of the nurses' contract. (Objectives 7 and 9)

_____ 38. One reason that nurses may not wish to be represented by other than their professional organization is the fear that their collective bargaining powers will be compromised. (Objective 9)

_____ 39. The National Union of Hospital and Health Care Employees now represents more nurses at the bargaining table than any other group. (Objective 9)

_____ 40. An important part of a contract is the section that establishes the grievance process. (Objective 10)

## MATCHING QUESTIONS

*Instructions: Match the numbered items with the most appropriate lettered items.*

### Group A (Objective 1)

_____ 1. Mission statement

_____ 2. Job descriptions

_____ 3. Chain of command

_____ 4. Channels of communication

_____ 5. Centralized organization

_____ 6. Decentralized organization

a. Patterns of message-giving within the organization

b. A statement outlining the purpose of the organization

c. The authority to make decisions is vested in a few people

d. Written statements that describe the duties and functions of the various jobs within the organization

e. Decision making involves a number of individuals and filters down to the individual employee

f. The path of authority and accountability from individuals at the top of the organization to those at the base of the organization

## Group B (Objective 4)

\_\_\_\_\_ 1. The case method

\_\_\_\_\_ 2. The functional method

\_\_\_\_\_ 3. Team nursing

\_\_\_\_\_ 4. Total patient care

\_\_\_\_\_ 5. Primary nursing

\_\_\_\_\_ 6. Case management

a. One nurse is assigned the responsibility for the care of each patient from the time the patient is admitted until that patient's discharge.

b. The nurse worked with one patient only and was expected to meet all the patient's needs, often living in the home and helping with household duties.

c. A nurse is assigned to a group of patients (4 to 6) and does all their care.

d. The nurse monitors an individual patient's health care from diagnosis through home care, assuring that the patient receives good and continuous care.

e. A group of variously educated nurses, each performing the tasks for which they were best prepared, care for a large group of patients.

f. Nursing tasks are assigned by the head nurse to various persons employed on the unit according to level of skills required for performance.

## Group C (Objectives 5, 6, 9, and 10)

\_\_\_\_\_ 1. Collective action division

\_\_\_\_\_ 2. Unfair labor practice

\_\_\_\_\_ 3. Agency shop

\_\_\_\_\_ 4. Lockout

\_\_\_\_\_ 5. Final offer

\_\_\_\_\_ 6. Grievance

a. Arbitrator selects the most reasonable package offered.

b. Requires those who do not want to be union members to pay the union fee rather than union dues.

c. A circumstance or action believed to be unjust or in violation of a contract.

d. Formed when a professional group assumes the responsibility for doing the collective bargaining.

e. Any action that interferes with rights of employees or employers in the bargaining process.

f. Occurs when the employer closes the plant to cause the employees to settle the contract.

## Group D (Objective 5)

\_\_\_\_\_ 1. Mediator

\_\_\_\_\_ 2. Union

\_\_\_\_\_ 3. Binding arbitration

\_\_\_\_\_ 4. Authoritative mandates

\_\_\_\_\_ 5. Collective bargaining

\_\_\_\_\_ 6. Common interest bargaining

a. Employer and employee representatives begin by identifying those areas in which they agree and those values and goals held by both parties.

b. An organized group of employees.

c. Employees who are members of the union participate in decisions with regard to employment, salaries, benefits, and working conditions.

d. Peaceful settlements encouraged by a high-ranking official.

e. Third person who joins bargainers to reconcile differences.

f. Both parties are obligated to abide by the arbitrator's decision.

## Group E (Objective 5)

\_\_\_\_\_ 1. No-strike policy officially adopted by the ANA.

\_\_\_\_\_ 2. First labor policy passed in the United States.

\_\_\_\_\_ 3. Taft-Hartley Act amends the NLRA.

\_\_\_\_\_ 4. Nurses are included in national collective bargaining policies.

\_\_\_\_\_ 5. ANA appointed a committee to study employment conditions.

a. 1935

b. 1945

c. 1947

d. 1950

e. 1974

# MULTIPLE-CHOICE QUESTIONS

*Instructions: Choose the one best answer for each question.*

1. Where do we find the broad goals of a hospital?

a. Articles of incorporation

b. Mission statement

c. Policy manual

d. Procedure manual

(Objective 1)

2. Mercy General Hospital is established to provide care to the abused and homeless in the community. Where would you expect to find this information?

a. In the hospital's job descriptions

b. In the minutes of the board meeting

c. In the channels of communication

d. In the statement of the hospital's mission and philosophy

(Objective 1)

3. What is the term applied to an organization in which the operation and administration is accomplished through a number of departments and subdivisions?

a. Autocratic

b. Bureaucratic

c. Canonistic

d. Democratic

(Objective 2)

4. Which of the following represents a central goal of most organizations?

a. To seek a structure that is efficient while providing maximum effectiveness

b. To seek a structure that allows everyone to have input into decision making

c. To seek a structure in which a wide margin of profit is assured

d. To seek a structure in which it is clear who is making decisions by virtue of the organizational chart

(Objective 2)

5. What is the term used to refer to the plan that describes reporting relationships in an organization?

a. Chain of command

b. Channel of communication

c. Clinical ladder

d. Span of control

(Objective 2)

6. Your first job as a registered nurse is in a community hospital headed by an administrator and a vice president of patient care services. There is a nursing supervisor for each shift and head nurse for each of the units—15 in all. What would be the term applied to this type of structure?

   a. Centralized

   b. Decentralized

   c. Flat

   d. Nonhierarchial

   (Objective 2)

7. What is an alternate term that can be used to refer to the chain of command?

   a. Channel of communication

   b. Description of job

   c. Organizational hierarchy

   d. Protocols

   (Objective 2)

8. Properly employed, the channels of communication within an organization typically reflect which of the following?

   a. Centralization pattern

   b. Job descriptions

   c. Lines of authority

   d. Span of control

   (Objective 2)

9. As a staff nurse you accept the assignment to provide the care to six patients on a surgical unit. Which of the following best describes this arrangement?

a. You have authority for this assignment.

b. It becomes your responsibility.

c. It is an example of cross-training.

d. There is little accountability attached to the assignment.

(Objective 2)

10. You are working in a staffing situation in which nursing teams are composed of one registered nurse and one nursing assistant. You assign the nursing assistant on your team to do vital signs on all patients. Which of the following is true of this situation?

    a. The nursing assistant is solely accountable for the care.

    b. It is the responsibility of the head nurse to check that the nursing assistant competes this assignment.

    c. No one is responsible; it's a basic expectation of the situation.

    d. You are accountable for the care you have delegated to the nursing assistant.

    (Objective 2)

11. You are interested in learning more about organizations and decide to review the job description for the staff nurse in your hospital. Where are you most likely to find this document?

    a. In the mission statement

    b. In the procedure book

    c. In the policy manual

    d. In the board manual

    (Objective 2)

12. In addition to describing the duties and functions of various jobs within the organization, which of the following does a job description also define?

    a. The salary to be earned in that position

    b. The process of evaluation to be used

c. The cross-training involved

d. The scope of authority, responsibility, and accountability for each position

(Objective 2)

13. Which of the following is the term we apply to a situation in which one member of the health care team performs functions usually associated with another position?

    a. Cross-training

    b. Delegating

    c. Economizing

    d. Self-directing

    (Objective 2)

14. As a new graduate, you are not absolutely certain how to proceed with a certain treatment and wish to be assured you are knowledgeable before beginning the care. Where are you most likely to find the information you need?

    a. In the hospital's job descriptions

    b. In the hospital's policy manual

    c. In the hospital's procedure manual

    d. In the hospital's standards of care

    (Objective 2)

15. If you are working in a hospital employing a shared governance practice model, which of the following would you expect?

    a. Nursing staff will be allowed to have input to major decisions within the organization.

    b. Nursing staff will have little input to major decisions within the organization.

    c. Nursing staff will have input into major decisions regarding the operation of their unit.

    d. Nursing staff will rotate through an Administrative Council where major decisions are made.

    (Objective 3)

16. Which of the following is often paired with a shared governance model?

    a. Case management

    b. Computer-assisted charting

    c. Team conferences

    d. Total quality improvement

    (Objective 3)

17. In which pattern of care delivery is each person responsible for specific tasks?

    a. Functional nursing

    b. Primary nursing

    c. Team nursing

    d. Total patient care

    (Objective 4)

18. In which pattern of care delivery is the nurse responsible for the patients' care 24 hours a day from admission through discharge?

    a. Functional nursing

    b. Primary nursing

    c. Team nursing

    d. Total patient care

    (Objective 4)

19. Within your nursing team, you assign the care of an uncomplicated postsurgical patient to the licensed practical nurse. Which of the following terms does this describe?

    a. Communicating

    b. Delegating

    c. Evaluating

    d. Processing

    (Objective 4)

20. Which of the following is the term used for a plan that allows the staff nurse to be promoted without leaving patient care?

a. Career pathway

b. Clinical ladder

c. Cross-training

d. Shared governance

(Objective 4)

21. What does the term *negotiate* imply?

    a. That labor can eventually "make a point"

    b. That management has the "upper hand"

    c. That mediation will be needed to settle the contract

    d. That there will be compromise by both sides

    (Objectives 5 and 6)

22. During which year was the Taft-Hartley Act amended to allow nurses in nonprofit hospitals to bargain collectively for salaries and working conditions?

    a. 1935

    b. 1945

    c. 1947

    d. 1974

    (Objective 5)

23. The Taft-Hartley Act is also known as which of the following?

    a. Wagner Act

    b. Labor Management Act

    c. NLRA

    d. Public Law 93-360

    (Objective 5)

24. Which of the following represents one of the reasons why nurses were not included in collective bargaining laws?

    a. Concern for the image of nursing

    b. The effect on physicians

c. The effect on health care

d. The cost to nurses

(Objectives 5 and 7)

25. What is the role of the person chosen by agreement of both parties to decide a dispute between them?

    a. Arbitrator

    b. Board of inquiry

    c. Conciliator

    d. Mediator

    (Objective 6)

26. When a branch of a professional association does the negotiating for its members, what is the name by which the group may be known?

    a. A union

    b. A closed shop

    c. An agency shop

    d. A collective action division

    (Objectives 5 and 7)

27. Why is an agency shop considered desirable by the employees' group?

    a. It encourages membership in the organization.

    b. It means higher salaries.

    c. It eliminates the cost of arbitration.

    d. It guarantees acceptance of the contract.

    (Objectives 5 and 7)

28. What is the implication of binding arbitration for both sides?

    a. Both sides are obligated to abide by the decision of the arbitrator.

    b. Both sides may make one final best offer.

    c. Both sides can bring new negotiators to the table.

d. Both sides have 10 days to settle their differences.

(Objective 6)

29. Which of the following makes a contract stronger?

    a. If it is negotiated each year

    b. If it is recorded in the county court-house

    c. If it is reviewed by an arbitrator

    d. If it is written

    (Objective 7)

30. In addition to other items, which of the following is included in a good contract?

    a. A copy of the bylaws governing the organization

    b. A section establishing guidelines for disciplinary problems

    c. The names of the chief officers of each party

    d. A copy of Public Law 93-360

    (Objective 7)

31. Which of the following represents one of the advantages of having nurses negoti-ate for nurses?

    a. They are a strong union.

    b. They have been doing negotiations for years.

    c. They have more funds to devote to the activities.

    d. They thoroughly understand the concerns of nurses.

    (Objective 9)

32. Which of the following represents one argument for having another organiza-tion do the negotiating for nurses?

    a. It is less expensive in the long run.

    b. Another organization may understand the nuances of bargaining better than nurses.

c. It will help avoid strikes and, therefore, interruption of care.

d. It will create and maintain a better image for nurses.

(Objective 9)

33. Which of the following best explains concession bargaining?

    a. A process by which there is an explicit exchange of labor cost for improve-ments in job security

    b. A process by which each party gives in on critical issues

    c. A process by which management offers compromises to the union in exchange for longer hours

    d. A process by which the union requests additional pay for longer hours

    (Objectives 5 and 6)

34. Which of the following represents one of the recent controversial issues related to collective bargaining in nursing?

    a. The makeup of the negotiating team

    b. The involvement of the staff nurse in the contract development process

    c. The distinguishing between profession-al knowledge and front-line manager duties

    d. The fees charged by the professional negotiators to the organization they represent

    (Objective 8)

35. Which organization represents the major-ity of nurses at the bargaining table?

    a. Federation of Nurses and Health Care Professionals

    b. National League for Nursing

    c. State nurses' association

    d. Teamsters

    (Objective 9)

36. What is the purpose of a grievance process in a contract?

    a. Differentiate grievances from complaints

    b. Protect the "little guy"

    c. Establish a method for adjustment of grievances

    d. Protect the management from "wrongful suits"

    (Objective 10)

37. In what way is a grievance different than a complaint?

    a. A grievance costs the employee dollars, a complaint does not.

    b. A grievance must relate to assigned work hours, complaints are broader.

    c. A complaint is a circumstance believed to be in violation of the contract, a grievance relates to working conditions.

    d. A grievance represents a circumstance believed to be in violation of the contract, a complaint is not.

    (Objective 10)

38. Which of the following is characteristic of the grievance process?

    a. It is typically cumbersome and difficult to implement.

    b. It typically involves a series of steps accompanied by time lines.

    c. It eventually requires input from a mediator.

    d. It is to be avoided if at all possible because of the large amount of time it takes.

    (Objective 10)

39. Which of the following is a recent activity initiated by the ANA to improve the work environment?

    a. Providing financial assistance to all state nurses' associations to assist them with collective bargaining activities.

    b. Requiring through the JCAHO that security persons be employed in all emergency rooms.

    c. Providing tuition-free courses to all hospital supervisors on workplace safety.

    d. Providing money to selected states to initiate or improve workplace advocacy programs.

    (Objective 9)

40. What has been the impact of shared governance on the collective bargaining process?

    a. Many of the issues are now resolved at the committee or council level.

    b. The role of the supervisor has become more blurred.

    c. It has lessened the accountability of the staff nurse in the process.

    d. It has made collective bargaining totally unnecessary.

    (Objectives 7 and 8)

## GAMING IN THE CLASSROOM

*Instructions: This game involves selecting teams and a host. The teams compete against one another for points. Each game has several subject categories. After teams are determined, a team is chosen to go first and selects a category. The host then poses the answer and the team provides the correct question for that answer. Each question can be awarded the same number of points or more difficult questions may be given heavier point values. (The instructor might determine which questions are more difficult based on the content emphasized in class.) Points are awarded to the team that is the first to signal and give a correct question. If that team is incorrect, the other team may attempt to provide the correct question and receive the points. The length of time allowed for response can be determined by the class or by the instructor. The team with the most points at the end of the game is declared the winner. Teams may be composed of individual students or groups of students. Teams may determine their answers as a team or may take turns answering as individuals.*

## Categories

A. Terms Used in Hospital Governance

B. Patterns of Nursing Care Delivery

C. History of Collective Bargaining

D. Collective Bargaining Terminology

E. Nursing Issues and Collective Bargaining

## Answers and Questions

### Category A

A: Outlines the goals and purposes of an organization.

Q: What is a mission statement?

A: Is a graphic, pictorial means of portraying various roles and patterns of interaction among parts of a system.

Q: What is an organizational chart?

A: Refers to the number of employees supervised by a manager.

Q: What is the span of control?

A: The path of authority and accountability from individuals at the top of the organization to those at the base.

Q: What is the chain of command?

A: Patterns of message giving within an organization?

Q: What are channels of communication?

### Category B

A: The first system used for the delivery of nursing care in the United States.

Q: What is the case method?

A: One nurse might take all temperatures, another do all dressings, while another administers all medications and charts them.

Q: What is the functional method?

A: An important part of this form of nursing is a conference at which all the workers come together to plan patient care.

Q: What is team nursing?

A: An associate nurse is employed to carry out the plan of care when the assigned nurse has a day off.

Q: What is primary nursing?

A: Individual patient's health care is monitored for the purpose of maximizing positive outcomes and containing costs.

Q: What is case management?

### Category C

A: An individual who gave impetus to collective bargaining issues in his editorial column.

Q: Who was Horace Greeley?

A: The act that became the national labor policy of the United States.

Q: What was the National Labor Relations Act? (Or What was the Wagner Act?)

A: The American Nurses Association created an ANA Economic Security Program during this year.

Q: What was 1946?

A: Heavy lobbying on the part of hospitals excluded nonprofit hospitals from the legal obligation of bargaining with their employees.

Q: What is the Taft-Hartley Act of 1947?

A: The year the Taft-Hartley Act was amended to provide economic security programs for those employed in nonprofit hospitals.

Q: What is 1974?

## Category D

A: Implies a discussion of the terms of the agreement and suggests that there will be give and take.

Q: What is bargaining?

A: A legally authorized organized group of employees that negotiates and enforces labor agreements.

Q: What is a union?

A: An agreement between two or more people to do something, especially one formally set forth in writing and enforceable by law.

Q: What is a contract?

A: Any action that interferes with the rights of employees or employers as described in the amended NLRA.

Q: What is an unfair labor practice?

A: A third person who may join the bargainers in early sessions to assist the parties in reconciling differences and arriving at a peaceful agreement.

Q: Who is the mediator?

## Category E

A: Was at one time an issue with nurses but is not so controversial today.

Q: What is the issue of whether nurses should strike?

A: This federal act was tremendously influential in encouraging collective bargaining among nurses.

Q: What is the National Labor Relations Act?

A: Some would say that this is the most difficult issue facing nurses as they begin to bargain collectively.

Q: What is the issue of who will represent them at the bargaining table?

A: May be the most critical issue related to having a group other than nurses doing the bargaining for them.

Q: What is the cost of additional membership dues?

A: In 1984 the NLRB determined this issue would be decided on a case-by-case basis.

Q: What is the number of employee bargaining units that would exist within the health care industry?

# Answer Key

## CHAPTER 1

### Fill in the Blanks

1. length of stay, type of service, ownership
2. short stay, traditional acute care, long-term care
3. hospitals
4. months to years
5. 24 hours
6. a tertiary
7. transitional
8. proprietary or profit
9. 24 hours
10. step-down
11. public health department
12. medical treatment
13. 85 or older
14. assisted-living
15. continuing care retirement community
16. emergent
17. an ambulatory
18. bachelor's
19. symptom
20. resources
21. general, specialty
22. primary care provider
23. back manipulation, nutritional counseling
24. board certified
25. feet
26. ophthalmologist
27. master's
28. technologist
29. physician's assistants
30. rural, low economic
31. specialty
32. generalists, specialists
33. interdisciplinary
34. strength
35. physicians, nurses
36. warm
37. phytochemicals, antioxidants
38. chiropractic
39. lifestyle, diet, exercise, vitamins, herbs
40. client choice, informed consent, beneficence, nonmaleficence

### True-False Questions

1. T
2. T
3. F
4. F
5. T
6. T
7. T
8. F
9. F
10. F
11. F
12. F
13. T
14. F
15. F
16. T
17. F
18. T
19. F
20. F
21. T
22. T
23. F

24. T
25. F
26. F
27. T
28. T
29. F
30. F
31. T
32. F
33. F
34. F
35. T
36. F
37. F
38. T
39. T
40. F
41. T
42. F
43. F
44. T
45. T
46. T

## Matching Questions

Group A
1. c
2. d
3. b
4. a

Group B
1. a
2. c
3. a
4. d

Group C
1. b
2. a
3. c
4. d

Group D
1. b
2. d
3. c
4. a

## Multiple-Choice Questions

1. d
2. a
3. b
4. d
5. a
6. b
7. a
8. d
9. d
10. a
11. d
12. c
13. d
14. a
15. b
16. b
17. a
18. a
19. c
20. d
21. b
22. a
23. c
24. d
25. a
26. c
27. c
28. c
29. b
30. d
31. a
32. b
33. b
34. c
35. a
36. b
37. d
38. c
39. a
40. d

# CHAPTER 2

## Fill in the Blanks

1. private payment, health insurance, charity care, governmental programs
2. third-party payer
3. Shriner's hospitals
4. 1930s
5. nonprofit
6. standards
7. Medicare, Medicaid
8. elderly, indigent
9. choice
10. skilled
11. evaluation
12. CHAMPUS
13. DRGs (diagnosis-related groups)
14. preferred provider organization
15. diagnosis-related group
16. prospective payment system
17. payment
18. controlling
19. fee-for-service
20. prospective
21. comorbidity
22. outlier
23. physician
24. complications
25. managed care
26. case management
27. vertically integrated
28. economic, geographic, sociocultural
29. economic, geographic, sociocultural
30. decrease
31. economically depressed
32. translators
33. JCAHO (Joint Commission, Joint Commission for the Acreditation of Healthcare Organizations)
34. HMOs
35. Utilization, Quality Control Peer Review Organization
36. critical path
37. physicians
38. regulatory
39. third-party payers
40. emergency room
41. key indicator

## True-False Questions

1. T
2. F
3. F
4. T
5. T
6. T
7. F
8. F
9. T
10. F
11. T
12. F
13. F
14. T
15. T
16. F
17. F
18. T
19. F
20. T
21. F
22. T
23. T
24. F
25. F
26. F
27. T
28. T
29. F
30. T
31. T
32. F
33. F
34. T
35. T
36. T
37. F
38. F
39. T
40. T
41. F
42. F

43. T
44. F
45. F
46. T
47. F
48. T
49. T

## Matching Questions

Group A
1. c
2. b
3. a
4. c

Group B
1. d
2. b
3. c
4. a

Group C
1. a
2. c
3. b
4. d

Group D
1. b
2. c
3. d
4. a

## Multiple-Choice Questions

1. a
2. b
3. b
4. c
5. b
6. d
7. b
8. b
9. a
10. c
11. a
12. a
13. d
14. a
15. a
16. b
17. a
18. c
19. c
20. d
21. c
22. d
23. d
24. c
25. a
26. a
27. a
28. c
29. d
30. c
31. b
32. a
33. a
34. c
35. a
36. c
37. c
38. c
39. b
40. b
41. a
42. c

# CHAPTER 3

## Fill in the Blanks

1. decision making, allocation of resources
2. organizations, government
3. financial
4. supplies, personnel
5. budget or authorization
6. ANA-PAC
7. voting, shaping public opinion, communicating with legislators
8. women
9. overview
10. American Journal of Nursing
11. legislators, legislative staff
12. elected representatives (senators/congressperson)
13. bias
14. vote
15. personal, form
16. restricted (limited)
17. N-STAT
18. PAC (political action committee)
19. ANA-PAC
20. Hatch
21. capital improvements, student assistance
22. Medicare, Medicaid
23. promote worker safety
24. promote health of mothers, infants, and children
25. authorization, appropriation
26. OBRA 87
27. state
28. Nursing Practice
29. Ontario
30. local
31. local
32. local
33. specialty
34. continuing education
35. state associations
36. ANA
37. supporting minority nursing students
38. support nursing education
39. consumers
40. NLN
41. CHAP
42. voluntary
43. Sigma Theta Tau
44. Fellow of American Academy of Nursing
45. ANA-PAC
46. Tri-Council
47. State Nurses Association
48. ANA-PAC

## True-False Questions

1. F
2. T
3. F
4. T
5. T
6. F
7. F
8. F
9. F
10. F
11. F
12. F
13. T
14. F
15. T
16. T
17. F
18. F
19. T
20. T
21. F
22. F
23. F
24. T
25. T
26. F
27. F
28. F
29. T
30. T
31. T
32. T
33. T
34. F
35. T
36. F

37. F
38. T
39. T
40. T
41. F
42. T
43. T
44. F
45. T
46. T

## Matching

Group A
1. a
2. d
3. c
4. b

Group B
1. d
2. a
3. c
4. b

Group C
1. b
2. a
3. d
4. c

Group D
1. d
2. a
3. b
4. c

Group E
1. d
2. c
3. a
4. b

## Multiple-Choice Questions

1. b
2. a
3. a
4. a
5. c
6. c
7. b
8. d
9. d
10. a
11. a
12. d
13. b
14. d
15. d
16. b
17. d
18. b
19. d
20. c
21. c
22. b
23. b
24. c
25. d
26. d
27. b
28. d
29. a
30. c
31. b
32. a
33. d
34. c
35. d
36. b

# CHAPTER 4

## Fill in the Blanks

1. priests
2. Egypt
3. punishment for sin, displeasing the gods
4. Greece
5. public hygiene
6. Siddhartha Gautama
7. China
8. Aztecs
9. folk, religious, servant
10. deaconesses
11. public health nurses
12. Fabiola, Marcella, St. Paula
13. Parabolani brotherhood
14. Rufaida Al-Asalmiya
15. change in the role of women
16. Protestant Reformation
17. Sairey Gamp
18. (Any two of) Order of the Visitation of Mary, St. Vincent de Paul, Sisters of Charity
19. Hospital of Immaculate Conception
20. Ursuline Sisters
21. Florence Nightingale
22. establishment of a school of nursing
23. Red Rover
24. Clara Barton
25. New England Hospital for Women
26. apprenticeship, workforce
27. Handbook of Nursing for Family and General Use
28. World's Fair, Chicago
29. Philadelphia, 1751
30. Benjamin Franklin
31. (Any of) a department of Pennsylvania Hospital; a hospital in Willamsburg, VA; or Friend's Hospital
32. Dorothea Dix
33. advances in medical science, the development of medical technology, changes in medical education, the growth of the health insurance industry, greater government involvement in health care, the emergence of professional nursing (any four)
34. Flexner Report
35. destitute elderly
36. Baylor University Hospital; Dallas, Texas
37. Hill-Burton Act
38. Social Security Act
39. (Any two) establish and maintain high standards of hospital service, care of the sick, control and prevention of disease
40. certified, skilled nursing facilities

## True-False Questions

1. T
2. T
3. F
4. F
5. T
6. T
7. F
8. F
9. T
10. T
11. T
12. F
13. F
14. T
15. F
16. T
17. F
18. F
19. T
20. F
21. F
22. T
23. F
24. T
25. T
26. T
27. F
28. T
29. F
30. F
31. T
32. T
33. F
34. T
35. F
36. F
37. F

38. T
39. F
40. T

## Matching Questions

Group A
1. c
2. e
3. a
4. f
5. b
6. d

Group B
1. e
2. d
3. c
4. a
5. b

Group C
1. c
2. d
3. f
4. e
5. a
6. b

Group D
1. d
2. e
3. b
4. a
5. c

## Multiple-Choice Questions

1. b
2. d
3. c
4. a
5. c
6. c
7. a
8. d
9. d
10. c
11. b
12. b
13. a
14. b
15. b
16. c
17. a
18. b
19. b
20. d
21. a
22. b
23. c
24. b
25. b
26. d
27. c
28. b
29. a
30. c
31. c
32. d
33. d
34. b
35. c
36. d
37. b
38. a
39. d
40. a

# CHAPTER 5

## Fill in the Blanks

1. technological advances
2. Florence Nightingale
3. medicine, nursing
4. medicine
5. nursing
6. Virginia Henderson
7. American Nurses Association, National Council of State Boards of Nursing
8. theoretical, practical
9. Flexner Report
10. body of specialized knowledge
11. scientific method
12. nursing research, nursing practice
13. education
14. autonomously
15. ANA Code for Nurses
16. International Code for Nurses
17. life work (or similar words)
18. giving away
19. professional
20. Public Law 93-360
21. levels of practice
22. restrictive
23. image of nursing
24. women
25. newspapers, magazines
26. public thinks about nurses
27. 1900s
28. The Educational Status of Nursing
29. supply and demand for nurses
30. placed in institutions of higher education
31. associate degree nursing programs
32. nurses and what they are doing
33. An Abstract for Action
34. 1979 Nursing Training Amendments
35. Pew Charitable Commission
36. pin
37. Maltese Cross
38. cap
39. uniform
40. pinning

## True False Questions

1. F
2. T
3. F
4. T
5. T
6. F
7. T
8. F
9. T
10. T
11. F
12. T
13. F
14. T
15. F
16. T
17. T
18. T
19. F
20. T
21. F
22. F
23. T
24. F
25. T
26. T
27. F
28. F
29. T
30. F
31. T
32. F
33. T
34. F
35. F
36. T
37. T
38. F
39. T
40. T

## Matching Questions

Group A
1. d
2. a
3. f
4. c
5. b
6. e

Group B
1. b
2. d
3. f
4. e
5. a
6. c

Group C
1. d
2. e
3. b
4. f
5. a
6. c

Group D
1. d
2. a
3. c
4. f
5. b
6. e

## Multiple-Choice Questions

1. a
2. b
3. c
4. d
5. b
6. c
7. d
8. a
9. d
10. d
11. b
12. b
13. a
14. b
15. d
16. a
17. d
18. a
19. c
20. c
21. a
22. d
23. d
24. c
25. a
26. a
27. b
28. d
29. c
30. a
31. c
32. b
33. c
34. b
35. a
36. d
37. a
38. d
39. c
40. b
41. c

# CHAPTER 6

## Fill in the Blanks

1. Omnibus Reconciliation Act
2. YWCA
3. 1940s
4. diploma
5. 1952
6. diversity
7. community-based experiences
8. 1909
9. research
10. Yale
11. licensure examination
12. registered nurse baccalaureate
13. standardized, validated
14. moving up the educational ladder, increasing their education
15. Education for the Future
16. NLN
17. institutions of higher education
18. baccalaureate degree
19. associate degree
20. North Dakota
21. scope of practice
22. grandfather
23. (Any of these) titling, interstate endorsement, grandfathering, scope of practice
24. interstate endorsement
25. competencies
26. licensing examination
27. educational mobility
28. community-based
29. computers
30. theories
31. adaptation
32. systems
33. Martha Rodgers
34. self-care
35. Virginia Henderson
36. interpersonal
37. continuing education
38. Teachers College, Columbia University
39. continuing education units
40. current in practice (or similar words)

## True-False Questions

1. T
2. F
3. F
4. T
5. F
6. F
7. T
8. F
9. T
10. T
11. F
12. T
13. F
14. T
15. F
16. T
17. F
18. T
19. T
20. F
21. T
22. T
23. F
24. T
25. F
26. T
27. T
28. T
29. F
30. T
31. T
32. F
33. F
34. T
35. T
36. F
37. F
38. T
39. T
40. T
41. F
42. F
43. T
44. T
45. F
46. T
47. F

48. T
49. T
50. F
51. T
52. F
53. F
54. F
55. T

## Matching Questions

Group A
1. b
2. e
3. f
4. a
5. c
6. d

Group B
1. d
2. b
3. f
4. c
5. e
6. a

Group C
1. f
2. a
3. e
4. b
5. c
6. d

Group D
1. c
2. e
3. a
4. d
5. f
6. b

## Multiple-Choice Questions

1. c
2. c
3. b
4. a
5. b
6. a
7. b
8. b
9. c
10. a
11. d
12. a
13. c
14. b
15. c
16. d
17. d
18. c
19. c
20. c
21. b
22. b
23. a
24. d
25. b
26. a
27. a
28. b
29. a
30. a
31. c
32. a
33. a
34. c
35. b
36. a
37. c
38. d
39. a
40. b
41. d
42. b
43. c
44. d
45. c
46. a
47. a
48. a
49. d
50. d
51. c
52. c
53. a
54. b
55. a

# CHAPTER 7

## Fill in the Blanks

1. protect the public, maintain high standards
2. accreditation
3. NLN
4. written
5. legal credential
6. state, professional organizations
7. nongovernmental
8. independent entity
9. Associated Alumnae of the United States and Canada
10. Permissive
11. New York
12. mandatory
13. mandatory
14. continuing education
15. ANA
16. baccalaureate
17. Associated Alumnae of the United States and Canada
18. state board of nursing
19. performing services for compensation, specialized knowledge base, use of the nursing process
20. rules, regulations
21. ANA, NCSBN
22. rules, regulations
23. State Board of Nursing
24. disciplinary action
25. approved
26. advisory opinion
27. appointed
28. NCLEX-RN
29. NCLEX-PN
30. adaptive
31. assessment, analysis, planning, implementation, evaluation
32. safe, effective care environment; physiological integrity; psychosocial integrity; health promotion/health maintenance
33. endorsement
34. must meet
35. adaptive testing
36. suspension, revocation
37. disciplinary action
38. attorney
39. substance abuse, commission of a felony, harming the public, fraud in obtaining a license
40. suspension, revocation
41. prevent exploitation of foreign nurses, help ensure safety of the public
42. American Nurses Credentialing Center, the AACCN (also AWHONN and others)
43. master's degree
44. simulation
45. standardized, accountable, flexible, effective, efficient

## True-False Questions

1. T
2. F
3. T
4. T
5. F
6. T
7. T
8. T
9. T
10. F
11. F
12. F
13. F
14. F
15. T
16. T
17. F
18. F
19. T
20. F
21. F
22. T
23. T
24. T
25. T
26. F
27. T
28. T
29. F
30. F
31. F
32. T

33. F
34. F
35. T
36. T
37. F
38. T
39. T
40. F
41. F
42. T
43. T

## Matching Questions

Group A
1. b
2. c
3. d
4. a
5. e

Group B
1. e
2. b
3. a
4. c
5. d

## Multiple-Choice Questions

1. a
2. d
3. c
4. a
5. c
6. a
7. b
8. d
9. a
10. c
11. a
12. c
13. c
14. c
15. d
16. c
17. b
18. a
19. a
20. c
21. a
22. a
23. b
24. b
25. c
26. d
27. b
28. d
29. d
30. a
31. b
32. c
33. d
34. b
35. d
36. b

# CHAPTER 8

## Fill in the Blanks

1. ethics
2. Law
3. enacted
4. statutory
5. criminal
6. common
7. civil
8. tort
9. crime
10. common
11. policy manual
12. nursing textbook
13. report
14. crime
15. civil
16. a license
17. legal authorities
18. respondeat superior
19. charitable immunity
20. nonprofit
21. delegating
22. claims occurred
23. claims brought
24. Liability insurance
25. volunteer
26. defamation of character
27. false imprisonment
28. confidentiality
29. competent
30. voluntary, informed
31. legal guardian
32. negligence
33. harm, duty, breach of duty, breach of duty is the cause of harm
34. malpractice
35. critical
36. use good interpersonal skills
37. deposition
38. discovery
39. Privilege
40. expert

## True-False Questions

1. F
2. F
3. T
4. T
5. T
6. F
7. F
8. F
9. F
10. F
11. T
12. T
13. F
14. F
15. T
16. T
17. T
18. F
19. T
20. T
21. F
22. F
23. T
24. F
25. T
26. T
27. F
28. F
29. F
30. T
31. T
32. T
33. T
34. T
35. T
36. T
37. F
38. F
39. F
40. T
41. F

## Matching Questions

Group A
1. f
2. c
3. e
4. d
5. a
6. b

## Multiple-Choice Questions

1. b
2. c
3. d
4. b
5. a
6. c
7. c
8. b
9. d
10. b
11. a
12. b
13. a
14. c
15. a
16. b
17. b
18. b
19. b
20. b
21. d
22. b
23. c
24. b
25. c
26. b
27. a
28. b
29. d
30. c
31. c
32. d
33. a
34. b
35. b

36. d
37. a
38. d
39. c
40. a

# CHAPTER 9

## Fill in the Blanks

1. moral
2. values
3. Values clarification
4. rights
5. rights
6. autonomy
7. beneficence
8. nonmaleficence
9. justice
10. fidelity
11. veracity
12. standard of best interest
13. paternalism
14. ethical theory
15. utilitarianism
16. social justice
17. natural law
18. Code for Nurses, International Council Code for Nurses
19. Patients' Bill of Rights
20. judicial system
21. funding
22. collegial
23. authoritarian, paternalistic
24. ethics
25. identifying, clarifying
26. solution  (or similar word)
27. commitment
28. slander
29. information (or similar word)
30. authority, responsibility
31. excellence
32. self-evaluation
33. pilfering
34. quality assurance
35. complete, appropriate
36. outcome criteria
37. Joint Commission for the Accreditation of Healthcare Organizations or Medicare
38. chemically impaired professional
39. from the hospital supply (or similar words)
40. know what the law in your state requires

## True-False Questions

1. T
2. T
3. F
4. F
5. T
6. T
7. F
8. T
9. T
10. T
11. F
12. F
13. T
14. T
15. F
16. T
17. F
18. F
19. F
20. F
21. F
22. F
23. F
24. T
25. T
26. F
27. T
28. F
29. F
30. T
31. T
32. F
33. T
34. F
35. T
36. T
37. T
38. T
39. F
40. F

## Matching Questions

Group A
1. d
2. f
3. a
4. b
5. e
6. c

Group B
1. e
2. a
3. c
4. b
5. d

Group C
1. f
2. c
3. a
4. e
5. b
6. d

Group D
1. d
2. f
3. e
4. c
5. a
6. b

## Multiple-Choice Questions

1. a
2. b
3. c
4. d
5. d
6. c
7. a
8. b
9. b
10. d
11. d
12. d
13. a
14. c
15. b
16. d
17. c
18. b
19. d
20. a
21. c
22. d
23. c
24. a
25. a
26. d
27. b
28. d
29. c
30. d
31. a
32. b
33. a
34. b
35. c
36. d
37. d
38. c
39. b

# CHAPTER 10

## Fill in the Blanks

1. Bioethics
2. center for research
3. technological advances
4. 1995
5. prevents conception
6. 1965
7. age of consent
8. emancipated minor
9. American Academy of Pediatrics
10. therapeutic
11. elective
12. Roe vs. Wade
13. amniocentesis
14. wrongful birth
15. eugenics
16. positive eugenics
17. genome
18. surrogate motherhood
19. 1978
20. homologous
21. Black's Law Dictionary
22. futile
23. Patient Self-Determination Act
24. living will
25. good death
26. negative, passive
27. positive, active
28. negative
29. competent, incompetent
30. Code for Nurses
31. negative right simpliciter
32. procurement
33. scarce medical resources
34. lack of education, information
35. xenotransplantation
36. acceptable behavior
37. pharmacologic agents
38. electroconvulsive therapy
39. rationing
40. cost, expense, or a similar word

## True-False Questions

1. T
2. F
3. T
4. F
5. T
6. F
7. T
8. T
9. T
10. F
11. T
12. F
13. F
14. T
15. T
16. F
17. F
18. T
19. F
20. F
21. T
22. T
23. F
24. T
25. F
26. F
27. T
28. F
29. F
30. F
31. F
32. T
33. T
34. T
35. F
36. F
37. T
38. F
39. T
40. T

## Matching Questions

Group A
1. c
2. d
3. e
4. a
5. b

Group B
1. d
2. c
3. a
4. b

Group C
1. d
2. a
3. e
4. b
5. f
6. c

Group D
1. c
2. a
3. f
4. e
5. b
6. d

## Multiple-Choice Questions

1. b
2. a
3. d
4. c
5. c
6. d
7. a
8. d
9. b
10. d
11. a
12. c
13. d
14. d
15. b
16. c
17. a
18. b
19. c
20. d
21. a
22. d
23. b
24. b
25. a
26. b
27. d
28. b
29. c
30. c
31. b
32. a
33. a
34. c
35. c
36. d
37. d
38. a
39. d
40. b

# CHAPTER 11

## Fill in the Blanks

1. hospitals
2. outside
3. outside the hospital
4. growing
5. greater
6. NCSBN
7. educational councils
8. criticality
9. (three of the following) theoretical background, nursing process, recognize own abilities and limitations, use communication skills, documentation, commitment to a work ethic, proficiency in technical skills, acceptable speed
10. universal precautions
11. assessment, analysis, planning, implementation, evaluation
12. abilities, limitations
13. coworkers
14. work ethic
15. functional
16. clinical
17. self-assessment
18. 5 to 10
19. learning
20. continuing education
21. 4
22. references
23. active
24. skills
25. feelings that result from feeling unable to meet expectations and powerless to effect changes
26. unrealistic
27. push themselves to the limit, give up values and standards
28. assertive
29. possible
30. chronic stress
31. physiological, psychological
32. ideals, reality
33. nursing staff, supervisory personnel, and hospital administration
34. Men

35. comparable worth
36. sexual harassment
37. telling the person
38. employer
39. personal awareness
40. needle-stick injuries
41. standard precautions (body substance precautions)
42. health, social service
43. assessment, analysis, plan

## True-False Questions

1. T
2. T
3. T
4. T
5. F
6. T
7. F
8. T
9. T
10. F
11. T
12. F
13. T
14. F
15. F
16. T
17. T
18. F
19. F
20. T
21. T
22. T
23. T
24. F
25. F
26. F
27. T
28. F
29. T
30. F
31. F
32. T
33. T
34. T

35. T
36. T
37. T
38. F
39. T
40. T
41. F
42. F
43. T
44. T
45. T
46. F
47. T
48. T

31. d
32. d
33. a
34. b
35. d
36. c
37. b
38. a
39. d
40. b

## Multiple-Choice Questions

1. a
2. a
3. d
4. a
5. b
6. b
7. b
8. b
9. a
10. c
11. d
12. c
13. a
14. b
15. c
16. d
17. c
18. d
19. a
20. a
21. a
22. a
23. d
24. c
25. b
26. b
27. d
28. c
29. a
30. b

# CHAPTER 12

## Fill in the Blanks

1. mission statement
2. division of labor
3. organizational chart
4. span of control
5. chain of command
6. channels of communication
7. responsibility
8. job descriptions
9. cross-training
10. clinical ladder
11. procedure manual
12. standards of care
13. shared governance
14. councilar, congressional, administrative
15. case method
16. functional method
17. team conference
18. team
19. primary
20. case management
21. delegation
22. negotiating
23. 1974
24. election
25. Horace Greeley
26. Wagner
27. Taft-Hartley Act, Labor Management Relations Act
28. common interest bargaining
29. collective action division
30. unfair labor practice
31. encourages membership in the union
32. binding arbitration
33. impasse, deadlocked
34. the cost involved or that it may result in a contract with which neither party is really pleased
35. financial remuneration, nonfinancial rewards, guidelines for grievances
36. professional
37. strike
38. concession bargaining
39. writing, resolve
40. grievance

## True-False Questions

1. T
2. F
3. T
4. F
5. T
6. F
7. T
8. F
9. T
10. F
11. T
12. F
13. F
14. F
15. T
16. T
17. F
18. T
19. F
20. T
21. T
22. F
23. T
24. F
25. F
26. F
27. T
28. F
29. T
30. T
31. T
32. T
33. F
34. F
35. F
36. T
37. F
38. T
39. F
40. T

## Matching Questions

Group A
1. b
2. d
3. f
4. a
5. c
6. e

Group B
1. b
2. f
3. e
4. c
5. a
6. d

Group C
1. d
2. e
3. b
4. f
5. a
6. c

Group D
1. e
2. b
3. f
4. d
5. c
6. a

Group E
1. d
2. a
3. c
4. e
5. b

## Multiple-Choice Questions

1. b
2. d
3. b
4. a
5. a
6. a
7. c
8. c
9. b
10. d
11. c
12. d
13. c
14. a
15. a
16. d
17. a
18. b
19. b
20. b
21. d
22. d
23. b
24. c
25. a
26. d
27. a
28. a
29. d
30. b
31. d
32. b
33. a
34. c
35. c
36. a
37. d
38. b
39. d
40. a